THIRD EYE AWAKENING

Guided meditation to activate pineal gland, expand your mind power, Intuition, and Psychic abilities.

Table of Contents

Chapter one What is third eye awakening?

The most effective method to Open Your Third Eye

Man with his third eye open

Ever considered how to open your third eye, home to your "intuition?" Your instinct and higher astuteness wake up when this vitality focus is completely open and adjusted. Tragically, for a large portion of us, building up our third eye chakra and its capacities is trying, best case scenario, and may even now and again appear to be distant. Here are a couple of straightforward advances and suggestions to help.

4 Proven methodologies for arousing the third eye

To start with, we will portray the most significant rules that will assist you with building up your third eye.

Develop quietness

Cultivate the quiet of the brain, regardless of whether it's through reflection, simply sitting smoothly in nature, or being caught up in your preferred workmanship or game practice.

Why? Since third eye discernment hoists your faculties to increasingly unobtrusive levels. Some call it "the space in the middle of", mystic capacities, the domain of the undetectable. To have the option to tune in to the messages and data that gets through your third eye, you ought to be prepared to see the murmur of its insight. On the off chance that your psyche is occupied or boisterous, you may miss its primary message.

Sharpen your instinct

There are numerous approaches to develop your instinct. The third eye is the focal point of understanding, vision, and higher insight. So shouldn't something be said about getting to know your fantasies and their implications, maybe checking out at clear dreaming, becoming acquainted with how to peruse a horoscope or tarot cards? Find better approaches to intuit into your day by day life exercises.

Why? Since the third eye is the primary seat of more elevated levels of recognition and instinct. One approach to see it very well may be "phony it until you make it." at the end of the day, be interested, find out about these instinctive methods. In time, these generally recondite practices will show up increasingly natural, and you will acquire trust in your very own capacities.

You don't have to pay attention to this – really, the inverse is prescribed. Have a ton of fun, investigate, and above all, keep your brain and chakras open to plausibility and marvel.

Make each cell in your body stir and cheer!

A large portion of us have fiery squares and awkward nature just as vitality attacking propensities that keep us from getting to our full imperativeness, which drives us to feel depleted, dissipated, dull... even sick.

Fortunately doesn't need to proceed! Top of the line creator and widely acclaimed master on chakras, Anodea Judith, will uncover the key to improving your vitality framework, during a free virtual occasion facilitated by The Shift Network: Supercharge Your Chakra Practice: How to Heal Your Energy Centers and Unleash the Full Power of Your Life Force.

Sustain your inventiveness

Let your inventiveness stream uninhibitedly by concentrating on explicit exercises or allowing your creative mind to imagination. For example, start learning another craftsmanship or art; don't attempt to be great, simply let your motivation go through your hands and be fit to be amazed by the outcomes.

Why? Innovativeness is an effective method to relax your sane personality – you know, the psychological babble that remarks each progression you make to see whether it's set in stone, that will in general control each activity with a particular plan and planned result.

At the point when you quiet the piece of your mind that needs to be accountable for how reality ought to be and use your innovativeness to open up conceivable outcomes, your third eye limit has more space to unfurl and bloom.

Ground yourself to all the more likely take off

For the greater part of us, it probably won't be evident that so as to open our third eye capacities, we have to initially land both our feet on the ground. Likewise note the significance of opening up continuously, building solid establishments first that will enable you to have legitimate insight and decipher your extrasensory recognitions with however much clearness as could be expected.

Why? Since we have to have enough vitality going through our entire body and fiery framework to help a sound opening of inconspicuous channels of recognition. At the point when the third eye gets enacted, the data that comes through might show up rather abnormal, new, or just upsetting to the basic personality.

Being grounded and having enough vitality enables us to venture into unobtrusive elements of discernment. It can assist us with opening up unhindered and stay away from the basic negative indications of third educational, for example, feeling muddled or befuddled.

Opened eye in high contrast

The most effective method to practice your third eye chakra

We should investigate straightforward yet productive activities to help the opening of your third eye. Here's a rundown of practices that will give a lift to your instinctive vitality focus.

Exercise your instinct; it's the primary capacity of the third eye

Rest under the moon light and mirror; the moon light takes after the nature of light of your instinctive focus

Sustain quiet to hear the knowledge of the third eye; tune in, the third eye's sound is progressively similar to a murmur

Reinforce the vitality of your first chakra, just as your throat chakra; both are helpful grapples for opening the vitality of your third eye in ground-breaking and adjusted ways

- Divination rehearses
- Dream work, dream translation, clear dreaming
- Representations
- Guided contemplation, quiet reflection
- Allow your creative mind to free
- It couldn't be any more obvious, center around the space "in the middle of" things

- Be interested about emblematic implications, images around you in various societies and timeframes
- Cooperative with nature and the vitality of the components
- Appreciate innovative artworks
- Working with internal direction, soul guides
- Practice consideration
- Develop your mystic capacities

Don't hesitate to attempt to appreciate the investigation. It's the most ideal approach to get vitality streaming in the third eye all things considered.

Cerebrum and the third eye in human body

How does the pineal organ impacts the enlivening of the third eye?

Situated between the foreheads and simply over the eye level, the third eye is related with instinct and insight. In the human body, this vitality focus is customarily connected with the pituitary organ, just as the pineal organ.

Organs and chakras are personally related as they speak to various degrees of substantial capacities, the first being centered around the physical, the other on the inconspicuous vigorous level. The pituitary organ is viewed as the "ace organ" in the human body since it controls a large portion of different organs and their hormone creation.

Shouldn't something be said about the pineal organ? The pineal organ is situated in the mind, at a similar level as the eyes. Its association with the third eye chakra or Ajna in the Hindu framework has for quite some time been researched by yogic customs and current mysticism the same. They see this organ as a potential seat of the spirit and its advancement, a hotspot for magical encounters and extrasensory recognition or mystic capacities.

This organ is generally viewed as responsible for delivering melatonin and controlling our rest cycle and our sexual development. The manners in which it capacities is firmly associated with the cycles of light and murkiness.

How the pineal organ capacities

To suport your pineal organ and the enlivening of your third eye, this is what you can do:

Head outside and get loads of regular light.

Eat nourishments or enhancements that help a sound action of the pineal organ (and counter its calcification, for example, iodine, chlorella, apple juice, Tamarind natural product (as it helps evacuate abundance of fluoride engaged with diminished pineal action).

Contemplate; reflection adjusts the action of the sensory system and invigorates portions of the mind that help the pineal organ.

Invest energy in complete haziness, as it invigorates a sound movement in the organ and creation of its related hormones.

Would you like to have more achievement and euphoria in your life? The most ideal approach to do this is by becoming familiar with your name through numerology. It is a multi year-old science that can assist you with learning the importance of your name, on the grounds that your name was no mishap! Everything necessary is your name and date of birth, click here to get your free customized numerology perusing.

Explicit practices to enact the third eye chakra

A reasonable and open third eye, otherwise called the Ajna, chakra encourages fixation, center, and dependence on instinct. Here are progressively explicit procedures for adjusting its vitality:

Simply Breathe

Careful breathing can quiet the psyche and, thusly, wash down and open the Third Eye. Being aware of your breathing takes into consideration purifying, yet in addition adjusts the chakra framework.

Include Third Eye Color

Related with the shading indigo, which is a blend of most profound blue and violet, the Third Eye chakra administers... Introduce blue and purple tones to your home and office stylistic theme. Encircle yourself with inconspicuous indigo tones can help mend the 6th chakra and lift vitality stream. Include valuable or semi-valuable blue-as well as purple-stone gems to your closet.

Practice third eye contemplation

Of the considerable number of activities you can accomplish for the 6th chakra, those that expect you to really draw in the Third Eye are the best.

Envisioning and ruminating over the shading blue or purple can help initiate the 6th chakra. For example, sit serenely and with eyes shut, envision a blue (or purple) chunk of vitality in the zone of your Third Eye. The Third Eye is critical in dreaming and dream review. Connect with and enact your Third Eye chakra by keeping a fantasy diary.

Work your theta brainwaves

It could be helpful to figure out how to initiate and keep up theta and alpha brainwaves. These encourage frontal flap action and set up your third eye and mind to be increasingly responsive.

Include some aroma

Acquaint basic oils with your home, shower, and body. Unobtrusive aromas can do some incredible things for opening, purifying, and adjusting the body's chakras. To help recuperate and initiate your 6th chakra, think about attempting one or a mix of these basic oils:

- Sandalwood
- Myrrh
- Roman or German Chamomile
- Grapefruit
- Nutmeg
- Eat (and Drink) Fruits and Veggies

Expending refreshments and nourishments with normal blue and purple tones can help support positive vitality move through the Third Eye chakra. Drink dull natural product juices, for example, grape and blackberry. Consider including the accompanying products of the soil to your staple rundown:

- dark currants
- blueberries
- blackberries
- eggplant
- prunes
- rainbow chard
- beets

Yoga for the third eye chakra

When figuring out how to open and recuperate the body's vitality focuses, no discussion is finished without presenting the advantages of yoga. The training's components of breath, center, and physical development, when taken together, are incredible apparatuses for purging and adjusting the chakras.

Step by step instructions to Awaken Your Third Eye

What is the Third Eye?

The pineal organ is a pea-sized organ molded like a pine cone, situated in the vertebrate cerebrum close to the nerve center and pituitary organ. Otherwise called the third eye, it is a worshipped instrument of soothsayers and spiritualists and viewed as the organ of preeminent all inclusive association. Its centrality shows up in each old culture all through the world. For instance, in Ayurvedic reasoning, the third eye is spoken to by the Ajna chakra and in Ancient Egypt, the image of the Eye of Horus reflects the situation of the pineal organ in the profile of the human head. The third eye is associated with clearness, focus, creative mind and instinct.

The Third Eye in Biology

The pineal organ speaks to the third eye in science, which produces melatonin. Melatonin controls circadian rhythms and conceptive hormones. This makes the pineal an ace controller of time, influencing our rest designs as well as our sexual development. Melatonin likewise influences our pressure and capacity to adjust to an evolving world. This third eye enacts when presented to light, and has various natural capacities in controlling the biorhythms of the body. It works in concordance with the nerve center organ which coordinates the body's thirst, hunger, sexual want and the natural clock that decides our maturing procedure.

Importance of the Third Eye

Building up the third eye is the entryway to everything mystic—clairvoyance, special insight, clear dreaming and astral projection. The dream of division among self and soul disintegrates when the third eye association is developed. Magical methods for being are associated with the third eye, for example, how to be wakeful inside the fantasy, to stroll among substances and outperform the restrictions of humankind.

Why You Should Awaken Your Third Eye

A blocked third eye or ajna chakra is said to prompt disarray, vulnerability, negativity, envy and cynicism. Through an open and lively third eye, the most elevated wellspring of ethereal vitality may enter. While the physical eyes see the physical world, the third eye sees the genuine world — a bound together entire with an unflinching association with soul. A rundown of the advantages and capacities the third eye brings incorporate clearness, focus, perspicuity, happiness, instinct, definitiveness and understanding. The third eye has been connected to clear dreaming, astral projection, nature of rest, upgraded creative mind and atmosphere seeing.

How Does Calcification Occur?

The calcification of the pineal organ is normal if the third eye isn't being utilized or because of diets wealthy in fluoride and calcium. Calcification is the development of calcium phosphate precious stones in different pieces of the body. This procedure happens on account of poisons in ordinary items, similar to fluoride, hormones and added substances, sugars and fake sugars. Radiation from mobile phone use and electric and attractive fields may impactsly affect the pineal organ also. Some connivance scholars accept broad communications crusades upholding the utilization of fluoride and calcium are spurred by government control programs.

Task: Celebrate the Third Eye

Most creatures have pineal organs, frequently bigger than human pineal organs, that drive instinctual information. While your pineal organ might be disregarded and decalcified, commend that you for sure have a pineal organ. Start your enactment practice essentially by sending appreciation to your third eye for your intrinsic instinctive capacities and your association with nature through the circadian rhythms that the pineal organ administers.

Go through 10 minutes every day deliberately initiating your third eye through contemplation, reciting, petition, move or yoga.

Third eye montage

Six Ways to Awaken Third Eye

Through decalcification and enactment, recover your way to happy euphoria and association with source:

Keep away from Fluoride

Give close consideration to the water in your life: faucet water is a wellspring of fluoride, which adds to pineal organ calcification. Fluoridated toothpaste is another conspicuous wellspring of fluoride in current weight control plans, as are inorganic produce and counterfeit beverages made with polluted water. Consider adding water channels to your sink and shower fixtures.

Supplement Your Diet

The rundown of enhancements that help and detoxify the third eye is long and incorporates crude cacao, goji berries, garlic, lemons, watermelon, bananas, nectar, coconut oil, hemp seeds, cilantro, ocean growth, nectar, chlorella, spirulina, blue green growth, crude apple juice vinegar, zeolite, ginseng, borax, Vitamin D3, bentonite mud and chlorophyll are generally fixings that helper filtration of the pineal organ.

Use Essentials Oils

Numerous fundamental oils invigorate the pineal organ and encourage conditions of otherworldly mindfulness, including lavender, sandalwood, frankincense, parsley and pine. Fundamental oils might be breathed in legitimately, added to body oil, consumed in a diffuser and added to bathwater.

Sungaze

The sun is an extraordinary wellspring of intensity. Look tenderly at the sun during the initial couple of moments of dawn and most recent couple of minutes of dusk to support your pineal organ.

Contemplate and Chant

Reflection initiates the pineal organ through goal: consider imagining the decalcification of the pineal organ, as its sacrosanct nature is lit up and straightforwardly associated with source. Reciting causes the tetrahedron bone in the nose to reverberate, which causes incitement of the pineal organ. Considering reciting "Om," otherwise called the sound of the universe, multiple times every day.

Work together With Crystals

Gems are powerful partners in the journey to stir the third eye. Use gems and gemstones in the purple, indigo and violet shading palette. This shading palette serves to stir, balance, adjust and sustain the third eye. Attempt amethyst, purple sapphire, purple violet tourmaline, rhodonite and sodalite. Spot the precious stone or gemstone between and marginally over the forehead during reflection.

Allow Your Intuition To sparkle

When you start working with your third eye, you will start to get direction messages and dreams. Endeavor to have the mental fortitude to finish on what your instinct offers and your third eye quality will just develop.

Third Eye Awakening: How to Recognize If Your Sixth Chakra Is Open

At the point when the third eye arousing occurs, there are some striking impacts on your reasoning and feeling.

The third eye (otherwise called the inner consciousness arranged between your eyebrows) is the 6th chakra with amazing capacities. Generally, this region or chakra becomes dynamic when the individual has arrived at a specific degree of mindfulness and awareness.

When that the individual has empathy, love, trustworthiness and duty, at that point the third eye opens and uncovers better approaches for self-advancement.

In the event that you need to know whether your third eye is conscious, here you have 4 signs that will assist you with remembering it:

1. Instinct

On the off chance that your 6th chakra is opened, the principal ability you will acquire is instinct. You will have the option to determine what, how or when something will occur before it really does. It is an unpretentious inclination that will manage you and which will grow more and better with time.

2. Diverse reasoning

You search for personal growth and you start embracing an alternate reasoning. You fire abandoning old propensities, old demeanor and you need a psychological and otherworldly advancement. You start pondering your life or life itself, you start addressing what you know or what you hear/see.

You start breaking down and scanning for better approaches for advancement – either society improvement or self-awareness. You never again acknowledge a variant of an answer, yet you look for reality and need to know more.

3. A receptive outlook

Your third eye arousing enables you to comprehend complex circumstances or ideas which before might have been unreasonably muddled for you. You start seeing a circumstance from numerous edges and you can comprehend its various perspectives. You are likewise ready to convey your emotions and considerations easily.

4. Seeing outside of the crate

Your reasoning is never again molded by what individuals or broad communications let you know. You see through words and you can get the genuine significance/purpose for activities. You are in contact with your faculties, with life, with nature and you can comprehend the concealed messages you get from them (for example synchronicity).

Chapter two How to awaken your third eye

Step by step instructions to Open Your Third Eye

In Hinduism, the third eye symbolizes a higher condition of cognizance through which you can see the world. Utilizing conventional reflection strategies, you can open up this chakra and addition a more profound, increasingly edified comprehension of the universe around you.

Find your third eye chakra. Chakras are the vitality focuses in your body. Basically, that are wheels of vitality that adjust along your spine. There are seven chakras, and each compares to an alternate piece of your physical, mental, and otherworldly prosperity. Your third eye chakra is the 6th chakra.The third eye chakra is situated at the bleeding edge of your mind, between your two eyes. It is directly over the extension of your nose. At the point when you ponder, attempt to concentrate your psyche on this chakra. It is liable for helping you to see the world all the more obviously.

Pick the correct environment. Contemplation is one of the best devices for helping you to open your third eye. By carrying more attention to your musings, you will have the option to all the more likely access the psychological clearness that is related with the third eye. The center objective of reflection is to expedite the psyche to rest one idea or item. It is critical to pick surroundings where you feel good when you are starting to meditate.A few people feel increasingly serene and liberal when they are out in nature. In the event that this seems like you, you should seriously mull over reflecting outside. Discover a space that is the correct temperature and where you can sit without being upset by others.

Indoor contemplation is additionally splendidly fine. Numerous individuals have an assigned reflection space in their home. This for the most part incorporates a pad that makes it progressively agreeable to sit on the floor, and maybe a few candles and calming music.

Recollect that contemplation is an individual procedure. You ought to pick the surroundings that are directly for you.

Set up your stance. The mind-body association is significant in contemplation. The more agreeable you are physically, the simpler it will be to concentrate on you contemplation item or thought. The best reflection pose is by and large idea to be some variety of sitting leg over leg on the ground. On the off chance that you are accustomed to sitting in a seat, take some time every day to become accustomed to sitting on the floor. In time, it will feel progressively common it will be simpler to concentrate on your contemplation. A great many people decide to use in any event one pad to make sitting on the ground progressively agreeable. Don't hesitate to utilize a few strong pads on the off chance that you discover this works better for you. On the off chance that you basically can't be open to sitting, don't stress. You can attempt what is known as strolling contemplation. For certain individuals, the cadenced hints of their footfalls can be exceptionally calming. Walk gradually, and have a make way with the goal that you don't need to ponder where you are going.

Pick a reflection object. A contemplation article can be an idea or a physical item. The purpose of picking one is to make it simpler for your mind to center. This will prevent your contemplations from meandering and will make your reflection more effective.Candles are a mainstream contemplation object. The gleaming fire is anything but difficult to take a gander at and are soothing to numerous individuals. Your contemplation object doesn't need to be close by physically. Don't hesitate to picture the sea or a lovely tree that you once observed. Simply ensure you can plainly observe the article in your inner consciousness.

Pick a mantra. A mantra is a word or expression that you will continue during your reflection practice. You may state the mantra inside or for all to hear - that is an individual inclination. Your mantra ought to be something that is close to home and significant to you.Your mantra ought to be something that you need to coordinate into your psyche, or your mindfulness. For instance, you may decide to rehash, "I pick satisfaction". This will help fortify the possibility that you are going to concentrate on feeling delight for the duration of the day.

Another mantra thought is to pick only single word. For instance, you could rehash "harmony".

Make it an everyday practice. Contemplation is a training. That implies that the first run through to plunk down to reflect, it probably won't be a major achievement. Your brain may meander, or you may even nod off. Figuring out how to effectively ruminate is a procedure and it takes time.

Make contemplation a piece of your consistently life. Start with exceptionally little additions, possibly five minutes or even only two. Before long you will feel increasingly good with the procedure and have the option to commit more opportunity to contemplation every day.

Realize being careful. Being careful implies that you are all the more effectively mindful of what is happening around you. You are intentionally focusing on your feelings and physical sensations. Being increasingly careful will assist you with getting on top of yourself and the world around you.As you are getting increasingly attentive, abstain from being judgemental. Simply watch and recognize without shaping a supposition about in the case of something is "correct" or "wrong".

For instance, on the off chance that you are getting a handle on pushed, don't pass judgment on yourself for feeling that way. Basically watch and recognize your feelings.

Head outside. Investing some energy outside can be extremely useful in getting progressively careful. Being progressively careful can assist you with opening your third eye since you will be increasingly mindful of it. Along these lines, it's a smart thought to attempt to go for a short stroll every day, with an end goal to invest more energy in nature.In the present culture, we are "connected" for quite a bit of our day. This implies we are quite often taking a gander at some kind of electronic or specialized gadget. Going outside reminds us to effectively take a break from the entirety of the improvements.

Be innovative. Being careful can enable you to get more in contact with your innovative side. Research proposes that careful reflection is an incredible remedy for author's squares and for hinders that craftsmen and other innovative sorts understanding. Being increasingly careful can enable you to open up your inventive pathways.Take a stab at trying different things with your innovative side. Take up painting, outlining, or learning another instrument. Letting your inventiveness stream will assist you with feeling more on top of yourself, and help you to open your third eye.

Concentrate on the little things. Everyday life can feel exceptionally chaotic and overpowering. Being increasingly careful can assist you with feeling quieter and better ready to use your third eye.

Focus on every part of your environment and your routine.For instance, when you are scrubbing down, deliberately watch the physical sensations. Observe how the warm water feels on your shoulders. Welcome the reviving aroma of your cleanser.

Feel progressively tranquil. When you figure out how to open your third eye, you will have the option to encounter the advantages that accompany it. Numerous individuals report feeling more settled subsequent to opening their third eye. Some portion of this is expected to accomplishing a more noteworthy feeling of self-sympathy. Being increasingly mindful of yourself by and large makes you practice progressively self-kindness.

Being kinder to yourself offers numerous advantages. You will feel progressively fearless and less restless. Be progressively learned. One reason numerous individuals need to open their third eye is on the grounds that it is thought to make you increasingly proficient. Since it expands your impression of your general surroundings, it bodes well that you will have the option to become familiar with your general surroundings. Individuals who have opened their third eye report that they sense that they have more wisdom.

You will likewise turn out to be progressively learned about yourself. Contemplation and care are extraordinary approaches to connect with yourself. At the point when you better comprehend your feelings, you will feel increasingly equipped for managing them.

Improve your physical wellbeing. Opening your third eye is probably going to lessen your feelings of anxiety. You will feel increasingly serene and mindful. There are numerous physical advantages from diminished degrees of stress. Individuals with less pressure are less inclined to have hypertension and indications of depression.

Encountering less pressure can likewise mean a decrease in things, for example, cerebral pains and upset stomachs. It can even assist you with having more youthful looking skin.

Third Eye Chakra Healing For Beginners: How To Open Your Third Eye

At the point when you initially catch wind of chakras, the idea can sound confounding. You may ponder precisely where all these chakras, including the third eye chakra, should be. In addition, how might we impact them? Do you need to turn into a contemplation ace to utilize them for recuperating? Therefore, you may feel enticed to simply proceed onward to another kind of mending work.

Nonetheless, opening chakras doesn't have to include long stretches of examining or practice. This manual for chakras for apprentices will concentrate on third eye arousing, specifically, investigating how you can recognize and evacuate squares to your third eye chakra. As it were, figuring out how to do third eye chakra practices sets you up for progressively complex chakra mending later on. This is on the grounds that the third eye chakra is tied in with sharpening your instinct and adjusting to the more extensive universe.

What Is a Chakra? Third Eye Chakra Meaning and Location

7-chakrasBefore we investigate how to know whether your third eye is open, it's critical to comprehend that the third eye chakra is one of seven individual chakras.

Running from the root chakra at the base of the spine to the crown chakra at the highest point of the head, every one of the seven chakras are amazing vitality focuses.

The point is to utilize chakra activities to keep all these vitality focuses open and adjusted. In the event that you can accomplish this, you'll be better ready to satisfy your maximum capacity and carry on with an upbeat life. Conversely, the more chakras are blocked or skewed, the more you'll detect something isn't right.

Third Eye Chakra Information Summary

Physical Location: In the focal point of your forehead.

Shading: Indigo.

Component: Extra-Sensory Perception.

Related Animal: Black Antelope.

Intense subject matters and Behaviors of Blocked Third Eye Chakra: When your Third Eye Chakra is blocked, you may battle to have confidence in your more extensive reason. In this way, you may feel there's no good reason for what you're doing, or feel it is inconsequential. You may likewise be struck by your powerlessness to decide. A few people depict this as a sentiment of mental loss of motion. On the off chance that you have a blocked Third Eye Chakra, you may experience difficulty resting, feel awkward, and battle to adapt new things.

Adjusting Chakras: What Is The Third Eye Chakra Responsible For?

The third eye chakra (or the Ajna chakra) sits between your foreheads, and it is associated with your otherworldliness, extensively translated.

Given the Ajna's significance, the third eye's parity influences (and is influenced by) the entirety of the accompanying things:

Your capacity to frame precise hunches.

Your feeling of the master plan throughout everyday life.

Regardless of whether you meet objectives identified with your most profound reason.

Adjusting feeling and reason.

Regardless of whether you feel you're dormant or pushing ahead.

In this way, when your third eye is open, you will utilize the two emotions and rationale to settle on critical choices throughout everyday life. You will trust in your very own instincts, and you will be happy with realizing that you're experiencing your motivation. At the point when you practice third eye chakra mending, you can see a significant distinction in your amends with your general surroundings, and on your capacity to be careful.

At the point when you're managing a third eye chakra blockage, you can begin to get negative third eye chakra indications. This can create when something makes you question your instinct's exactness, or when something gives you motivation to address what you thought was your motivation.

(For a large number of years, light specialists and vitality healers have utilized explicit stones to quiet and center the psyche, decrease pressure, and cultivate wellbeing and essentialness. Discover more and get your free vitality arm ornament, simply click here now to discover more...)

Manifestations of a Blocked Third Eye Chakra

Nobody experiences existence without pondering how to unblock chakras once in a while. Along these lines, don't stress if third eye chakra recuperating must be performed over and again.

The most significant thing is simply to have the option to recognize signs and manifestations of third eye chakra issues with the goal that you follow up on them as quickly as time permits. Here are the absolute generally normal:

- Absence of confidence in your motivation
- Feeling futile
- Hesitation
- Finding your work or life irrelevant
- Suspicion

Third eye blockages can likewise trigger a scope of inconvenient physical side effects. The most much of the time revealed include:

Cerebral pains (counting headaches)

Eye uneasiness

Back and leg torment

Sinus torment

Everybody has various triggers that sparkle the requirement for third eye recuperating. Be that as it may, it's valuable to know about the absolute most regular reasons for blockages in the third eye.

For instance, when somebody puts down your employment or enthusiasm, this can push the third eye chakra lopsided.

Likewise, experiencing a transitional beneficial encounter like sickness, passing, work misfortune or separation can make a blockage. Indeed, even simply moving into another period (for example around a huge birthday) affects your third eye chakra, given that it is so delicate to your view of your life's worth.

Third Eye Chakra Healing: How To Open And Unblock Your Third Eye Chakra

AjnaThird eye mending isn't as cloudy or mind boggling as it may sound. While the third enlightening experience can be significant, the kinds of systems that open the third eye chakra are shockingly straightforward.

We'll investigate four of the most helpful and clear approaches to gain by your new comprehension of the third eye's significance.

The entirety of the accompanying activities center around how to adjust your chakras, with an accentuation on the third eye chakra specifically.

In the event that you need some additional inspiration for utilizing and more than once rehearsing these strategies, simply recall that an unblocked third eye chakra can be the way in to a more joyful life. At the point when you have a finely tuned feeling of instinct, you normally float towards the open doors that are directly for you. What's more, monitoring third enlightening side effects is a simple method to tell whether you are living as per your actual reason.

1. Utilize Third Eye Chakra Stones And Jewelry For Healing

There is a chakra hues test that binds different various shades to various chakras. For the third eye chakra, the key shading is purple. This gives you helpful data to discovering third eye chakra stones to work with.

The idea is that you can discover adornments including purple stones and wear it whenever you have to unblock the third eye chakra. You can likewise buy bigger third eye gems that will sit in your pocket or in the palm of your hand, enabling you to crush them and spotlight on them when you have to keep your third eye chakra open.

Probably the best third eye stones incorporate the accompanying:

Purple fluorite: This semi-valuable jewel should elevate honed instinct and to clear up obfuscated contemplations. It's a perfect third eye chakra precious stone when you're attempting to settle on a troublesome decision and need to dispose of insignificant interruptions.

Amethyst: An acclaimed and lovely valuable stone, amethyst is customarily associated with third eye migraine help just as all types of mending. A few people additionally use it to speak to shrewdness.

Dark Obsidian: Another well known individual from the third eye precious stones gathering, dark obsidian advances balance among feeling and reason.

2. Third Eye Chakra Meditation And Yoga Techniques

Reflection may be one of the main things that rung a bell when you think about the inquiry "What is a chakra?". Notwithstanding, third eye reflection is only one of numerous approaches to take a shot at opening this chakra. Also, there are a lot of chakra contemplation methods for amateurs don't as well, stress on the off chance that you've never attempted care or reflection. Here's one to begin with:

Sit serenely and close your eyes. Breathe in and breathe out multiple times, gradually and profoundly. Concentrate on the area of the third eye chakra, envision a violet circle of vitality in your temple. Keep in mind, purple is the third eye chakra's shading. As you keep on breathing gradually and profoundly, picture the purple wad of vitality getting greater and hotter. As it does, envision it cleansing antagonism from your body.

Consider yourself of engrossing the third eye chakra's vitality—enable yourself to feel it everywhere.

Open your eyes when you feel prepared.

As you may have speculated, yoga can likewise be useful when figuring out how to adjust your chakras. Third eye yoga presents incorporate the youngster present and the bird present. You can discover pictures and recordings that will manage you through these clear positions. You may see third eye chakra opening side effects before long!

3. Chakra Foods List And Diet Suggestions

As is natural, fundamental chakra nourishments (for example ones that help all chakras) are for the most part sound staples. For instance, all organic products, vegetables, sound fats and wholegrain nourishments will in general advance transparency all through the chakra framework.

Be that as it may, there are additionally explicit third eye chakra nourishments, and adding them to your every day diet can anticipate or battle blockages. Remember the accompanying:

Dull chocolate: If you like dim chocolate, don't hesitate to have as much as you need when you're attempting to open the third eye! It is said to help improve mental clearness and lift fixation. It is an extraordinary wellspring of magnesium, which destresses you. As a little something extra, it advances the arrival of serotonin, placing you in a progressively positive disposition.

Anything purple: Given that purple is the third eye's shading, every single purple nourishment advance its equalization. The absolute best models incorporate eggplant, purple cabbage, red grapes, blueberries, and blackberries.

Omega-3: Foods that are wealthy in omega-3 can improve subjective capacity and along these lines help to keep your third eye chakra open. Great decisions incorporate pecans, salmon, chia seeds and sardines.

(Consideration: Energy mending searchers, get this mind blowing 'Reiki Energy Healing Bracelet' for nothing! Snap here now to get yours.)

4. Third Eye Chakra Affirmations To Use

Confirmations are phrases that target negative, restricting convictions and supplant them with increasingly positive convictions. They can be utilized to assist you including weight reduction to discovering love, so it makes sense that they can likewise be utilized to adjust chakras.

three-tips-for-making amazing attestations

When structuring third eye attestations, specifically, you need to concentrate on otherworldliness, your gut impulses, and your fundamental feeling of direction. Here are a few models you can attempt. Don't hesitate to change them until they feel right:

"I pursue the lead of my inward instructor."

"I realize how to settle on the correct choices, and I do as such effortlessly."

"I hear my instincts and I realize they will lead me to my motivation."

"I am on my actual way."

"I live each day as per my life's motivation."

"I confide in the direction that my third eye gives me."

"I have boundless conceivable outcomes accessible to me."

"I am an instinctive individual, and I realize what is directly for me."

"It is sheltered and great to pursue the direction of my third eye."

"My third eye is open and prepared to see my motivation."

Chapter three Best ways to open the third eye

Your third eye, or that 6th chakra that sits between your eyebrows and encourages you tap into your instinct in another manner, has been around for whatever length of time that you have. In any case, that reality alone doesn't mean you think a lot about it, including, on a fundamental level, what precisely it is. And keeping in mind that we're on the issue, you might need to realize how to open your third eye, correct? Fortunately specialists are here to clear things up—for the entirety of your eyes to see.

"The third eye is a vigorous focus, or chakra," says Erica Matluck, a naturopathic specialist, nurture professional, comprehensive mentor, and originator of Seven Senses, which encourages health withdraws. "Despite the fact that it's anything but a real physical structure, it is related with the pineal and pituitary organs on the mind and situated on the temple between the foreheads."

Matluck clarifies that the chakra framework resembles the organ arrangement of the inconspicuous (or fiery) body, and each chakra has a capacity or reason. The capacity of the third eye? To get to lucidity, instinct and prescience. "It enables us to see past what is physically present at the time," Matluck says. "Soothsayers and mystics normally have exceptionally grown third eye chakras."

"[The third eye] enables us to see past the what is physically present at the time." Erica Matluck, all encompassing mentor and naturopathic specialist

To that direct, figuring out how to open your third eye isn't something you can fundamentally achieve in an evening—it takes a mess of time and work, remembering putting a solid establishment for place. "Before we open the third eye, it is imperative to construct the lively establishment of the initial five chakras, beginning at the root (the first chakra)," Matluck says. "Endeavoring to open the third eye before working with the lower five chakras resembles figuring out how to bounce before you can even remain on two feet. Truth be told, opening the third eye rashly can bring about a profound emergency—regularly saw as psychosis."

At the end of the day, if opening the third eye is your definitive objective, it's an ideal opportunity to get the opportunity to chip away at unblocking and adjusting your different chakras (more exhortation on that here!). When you've done that, you can begin stepping toward opening that 6th chakra. Yet, recollect, this requires some serious energy—so show restraint toward yourself en route.

Need to realize how to open your third eye? The accompanying 11 hints can help.

1. Focus on your fantasies

Dreams can be befuddling, muddling, superb, and startling—yet don't simply disregard them every morning when your caution goes off. Seek them for help in opening your third eye. "Focus on your fantasies. Record them, recall them, and hear them out," recommends Matluck. Sounds like it's an ideal opportunity to air out that fantasy diary, huh?

2. Concentrate your contemplation on your third eye

Regardless of whether you utilize an application or practice care contemplation or supernatural reflection all alone, in case you're hoping to open your third eye, reflection can help with that a considerable amount. "Concentrate on the point between the temples in reflection, and essentially see what pictures or contemplations emerge," Matluck says.

3. Practice breath work

Breath work is a magnificent device to use in regular day to day existence, yet it's particularly useful in opening your third eye. "There are numerous sorts of breath work, yet holotropic breath work is especially appropriate to opening your 6th chakra," says Matluck.

4. Practice Kundalini yoga

In the event that you haven't attempted Kundalini yoga yet, pull out all the stops. The super-otherworldly (and regularly extraordinary) yoga practice is incredible for opening your third eye, particularly when you center around certain kriyas. "At the point when you practice Kundalini yoga, pick kriyas that emphasis on the pituitary or pineal organs," recommends Matluck.

5. Try not to surrender your ordinary yoga practice either

In the event that Kundalini is excessively scary or just isn't your thing, a standard vinyasa practice can assist you with figuring out how to open your third eye, as well. "One of my preferred postures for enacting the third eye is youngster's posture, with your temple squeezing into the floor," says Claire Grieve a worldwide yoga master, stretch specialist, plant-based wellbeing mentor. "Bring your center, consideration, and vitality into the chakra. Remain here for two to five minutes, inhale profoundly, and imagine your reality. Another extraordinary posture is forward crease: As you drop your head underneath your hips, blood and oxygen are raced to your cerebrum, and the third chakra conveys crisp vitality for arrangement."

6. Eat a nutritious eating regimen

Hate to break it to you, however opening your third eye isn't simple if all you're eating is lousy nourishment. This is on the grounds that your nourishment decisions are amazingly significant for chakra arrangement. "Your nourishment decisions administer your vitality," says Grieve. "Including a variety of purple nourishments, for example, blackberries, blueberries, grapes, eggplant, purple kale, purple sweet potatoes, and purple cabbage into your eating routine will lift and adjust your third eye."

She likewise noticed that nourishments like chlorella, spirulina, blue green growth, crude apple juice vinegar, chlorophyll, cilantro, crude cacao, goji berries, and nutrient D will assist you with detoxifying your pineal organ.

7. Start utilizing fundamental oils

Haven't taken advantage of your fundamental oil assortment in some time? It's a great opportunity to get moving, particularly if realizing how to open your third eye is the objective. Aromas like lavender, sandalwood, frankincense, white sage,

and pine can tenderly animate the pineal organ,"
Grieve says. "Utilize basic oils in the shower or in a
diffuser."

8. Reflect with precious stones

Precious stones are an incredible otherworldly
instrument to have in your back pocket—
particularly when you're opening your third eye.
"Have a go at setting a gem on your third eye as you
lay in an agreeable position and bring your
concentration into your breath," educates Grieve.
"Anything in the purple domain, for example,
amethyst, lapis lazuli, blue or purple sapphire,
purple violet tourmaline, or rhodonite will stir and
enact your third eye."

9. Have a go at tapping

Perhaps you've utilized tapping to help adapt to
pressure and tension. Indeed, the training is
additionally an extraordinary procedure for
opening the third eye. "Attempt tenderly tapping

the brow where the third eye is and initiating your pineal and pituitary organs by sending light floods of vibration," says reiki ace and culinary specialist Serena Poon.

10. Utilize sound recuperating

In the event that you've at any point gone to a sound shower, you think about the recuperating intensity of sound. What's more, solid is extraordinary for opening up your third eye, as well. "Utilizing sound recuperating or conditioning helps in contemplation and carries you to a theta state," says Poon. "This is a superb method to help open the third eye."

11. Work with reiki aces and different healers

The more work you put into mending yourself, the simpler it will be to open your third eye—so put in the work where you can. "Working with healers, accepting reiki and vitality work, and doing otherworldly advancement are on the whole amazing thoughts when you're opening your third eye," Poon says.

The Limitless Benefits of Opening Your Third Eye Chakra With Meditation: A User's Guide

Advantages Of Opening Third Eye

On the off chance that you needed to respond to the inquiry, "What number of eyes do you have?" and you replied, "Two, obviously!" that would be wrong. We really have three eyes, with the third eye being maybe the most dominant wellspring of information we have.

What is the third eye? In spite of the fact that undetectable, our third eye chakra is as present and accessible to us as our other two eyes.

What's more, here's a mystery you should know: It's a powerful wellspring of natural astuteness that when intensified with reflection, gives us understanding, cautioning and the most elevated conceivable degree of insight into the past, future, and above all, the present.

At that point, how would you open your third eye? What's the most ideal way?

Contemplation. Here is a short manual for see how to profit by your open and initiated third eye, and how and why contemplation is the best apparatus to get this going:

Third Eye Chakra Basic Questions Answered — #1:

What is the capacity of my third eye?

Advantages Of Opening Third Eye Chakra

For the most part known as the third eye chakra, this imperative, pineal organ found higher vitality field is the place we can take advantage of that which we can't see, taste, physically feel, hear, or smell.

This incredible "intuition" capacity rises above our five most fundamental human detects, for the most part making itself known to us by means of premonitions. It very well may be said that your third eye knows the obscure, sees the concealed.

With the developing acknowledgment of the bound together field hypothesis (that we are for the most part quantumly associated with each other), a developing number of researchers accept third eye instinct to be a legitimate, certain marvel.

Third Eye Chakra Basic Questions Answered — #2:

How would I know when my third eye chakra is open, stirred, and enacted?

Advantages Of Third Eye Chakra

Have you at any point gotten an inclination that somebody you love was in peril, and minutes after the fact, got a call to legitimize your sentiments? Have you at any point felt the compelling impulse to look behind you, and when you pivoted, your closest companion from secondary school was shopping in a similar market walkway? Do you ever consider somebody seconds before they send you an email or content?

The notorious saying, "all you have to know is as of now contained inside," is very valid and even (particularly!) down to earth in the present day and age. Furthermore, you can saddle and build up this capacity past levels you at any point thought conceivable.

Numerous exceptionally effective individuals owe, regardless of whether purposely or accidentally, their acclaim and fortunes to creating and believing the information got from their initiated third eye (making it no occurrence that such an incredible dominant part of fruitful individuals practice reflection).

Third Eye Chakra Basic Questions Answered — #3:

Things being what they are, do we as a whole have a third eye chakra?

Advantages Of Third Eye Chakra

Indeed. Despite your sexual orientation or strict (or nonreligious) conviction framework, we all have a special and possibly incredible third eye. The issue is, a considerable lot of current man's third eyes' are unactivated, "calcified", shut, lethargic, and unawakened.

The uplifting news? Reflection is the world's generally powerful and successful third enlightening, arousing, and decalcification apparatus.

You needn't bother with a precious stone ball. Hurl out your tarot cards. Disregard contingent upon a costly mystic to offer you the responses that you look for. All you have to know is as of now contained inside – open by means of your third eye. What's more, when you open it up this new measurement, get ready for an increasingly cognizant, significant, astute, and mindful life to unfurl.

Advantage of an Open Third Eye — #1:

Higher Consciousness - Zero Stress, Anxiety, Worry

Third Eye Meditation

With every session, contemplation normally moves your cognizance into increasingly elevated states, consequently discharging uneasiness and stress from every single present minute in your life (that implies consistently!).

Your pressure spiraling worries with how you are going to pay for your approaching home loan, understudy advance, and charge card bills will before long vanish, normally supplanted with irrefutable contemplations on the most proficient method to be fruitful to the point that the pre-reflection form of you appears to be ridiculous, sort of like glancing back at the individual you used to be in secondary school. Night and day.

All of a sudden, with an open and enacted third eye, everything comes into point of view, life's frequently unimportant stresses go to the wayside while you get an unmistakable image of your actual life reason — and how to satisfy it totally.

Third Eye Activation Benefit — #2:

Well honed Intuition: Harness The Wisdom Within

Opening Your Pineal Gland Chakra With Meditation

Similarly as reflection holds the advantage of arriving at higher conditions of awareness, enabling you to turn out to be progressively mindful, accomplishing authority of your feelings while effectively taking care of the pressure of your day, contemplation additionally tunes you into a characteristic conceived blessing we as a whole hold – natural astuteness.

Since numerous customary societies believe our instinct to be the most significant 'sense' or 'sight' in our ownership, third eye contemplation has been drilled for a considerable length of time.

As you contemplate and turn out to be increasingly more mindful of exactly how much purported inward knowledge you as of now have readily available, you'll need to keep opening and initiating your third eye to its fullest limit.

Incredible wellbeing? Your third eye instinct realizes how to reestablish. Better connections? Your third eye instinct realizes how to draw in. More profession and money related achievement? Your third eye instinct knows the bit by bit process. Knowing and satisfying your actual life reason?

Your third eye instinct knows correctly why you have picked this life as of now.

How much better would your life be if your save of inward unending shrewdness was available to your no matter what? Fortunately, contemplation is the absolute best arrangement.

Third Eye Meditation Benefit — #3:

Line up with the "Law of Attraction," Manifest the Life you Desire

Opening Your Eye Chakra With Meditation

We are altogether human, and keeping in mind that we as a whole need to have a dread free life, agonizing over how we'll achieve our day by day assignments, just propagates more stress. All things considered, as pulls in like, particularly valid with our musings.

In any case, when we set a period every day to rehearse contemplation, changing the idea of our considerations from the root, we start to have less and less stresses, tensions, and negative musings. Furthermore, when they go, what will have their spot will be more grounded and more on top of the ubiquitous law of fascination.

As your third eye opens to an ever increasing extent, your physical, mental, and passionate wellbeing duplicates, while new and more elevated level spirits start to normally enter your life — bringing about new and better connections on all fronts.

As your actuated third eye makes the right way to progress as clear and evident as the staircase prompting your second floor condo, contemplation will assist you with showing bounty as effectively and normally as relaxing.

Advantages of an Open Third Eye — #4:

To realize what's 'Out There', Look Inwards: Knowing The Best Path

Third Eye Meditation

On the off chance that you've at any point been keen on what hangs tight for you 'out there', yet you're not exactly sure what 'out there' is, know this present: it's not something to fear — dread need not have any significant bearing.

Any inquiries you have about your present life, for example, what work you should take, what decision you should make in your present relationship, or how you can achieve your greatest objectives and dreams, can be replied from the abundance of data contained inside during contemplation.

By initiating your third eye, contemplation enables you to see, comprehend, and appreciate the sights and hints of the recently shrouded world, enabling you to streamline and consummate your present life utilizing this huge hold of new data.

Become an accomplished eyewitness of the concealed, make the impossible...possible. Contemplation is the way to open your vast potential.

5 Signs Your Third Eye Is Openingthird eye

Since old occasions, the third eye had been loved by a wide range of societies. Today, we know it as the pineal organ, however it is still called the third eye in the profound domain. The third eye is seen as a profound sign speaking to our capacity to vanquish a wide range of difficulties in day by day life by taking advantage of our inward knowledge.

In any case, there is considerably more to the third eye than that. In most Eastern conventions, the third eye is without a doubt genuine; a thing that anyone can see and clearly feel on the off chance that they have a solid feeling of self and care. It is what is regularly alluded to as the association between our body and our soul.

At the point when we think with any consistency, the third eye opens and your internal guide becomes more grounded and an increasingly present managing power in your life.

HERE ARE FIVE SIGNS YOUR THIRD EYE IS OPENING:

1. A DULL SENSATION OF PRESSURE BETWEEN THE EYEBROWS.

By and large when the third eye begins to show on an a lot further level, there's a related awareness of sensation between eyebrows. It could appear as though someone is delicately contacting us right then and there, or you may feel a spreading of warmth.

Some of the time this sensation could show up from no place; regardless of whether we have profound emotions or not. Maybe it's a sign to pull us back in that otherworldly perspective.

2. Expanded FORESIGHT.

Among the most clear flag of third educational is an expansion in foreknowledge or instinct we begin to understanding – on the off chance that we are focusing.

Instinct is the ability to realize something may occur before it does or realizing something is correct or wrong due to an inclination or sense. It regularly goes back and forth without notice. Anyway with time, this inclination could get more grounded, and end up being a managing procedure in our every day lives.

We may begin to detect notice signs or what our next activity ought to be without clarification. Try not to question your instinct. Use it! It may not generally be correct; anyway it assuredly will put us on the correct way.

3. Inclined TO LIGHT SENSITIVITY.

With the opening third eye, we could get ourselves somewhat more delicate to light and seeing hues all the more brilliantly.

Distinctive hues and our attention to light may start unobtrusively; they are not in every case in a split second evident or overpowering. Be that as it may, the affectability to light regularly brings further familiarity with what's going on around us. When concentrating profoundly on the third eye (like in contemplation), the lights of the third eye may show up.

The third eye and it's reference to light has been discussed for a considerable length of time in numerous customs around the world. It is notable in numerous types of workmanship and strict works. In the event that you study the works, you can frequently observe the light reference in roundabout shapes and star-molded lights looking through the mists.

Our eyes will change after some time, and we may feel like we can't get enough sun on our skin. This is typical. Absorb it! Simply ensure you are not hurting the skin.

4. A FEELING OF GRADUAL AND CONTINUAL CHANGE.

Above all, cultivating a solid third eye consistently changes our point of view and character throughout everyday life. It brings about gainful changes since we need, and perhaps hunger for them. We can ordinarily observe it in the manner we treat others. We may turn out to be increasingly tolerant and less egotistical.

5. Expanded HEADACHES.

A cerebral pain pressure is more grounded than the weight discussed before that occurs between the eyebrows. On occasion, that weight can start to throb a bit. Think of it as a tad of vitality over-burden. Go outside and do a thing you love, as think or walk.

Head pressure is a real indication of the profound enlightening, especially in the focal point of the brow. It means that one's pineal organ is growing vigorously.

TIPS TO ENGAGE THE THIRD EYE

At the point when our Third Eye is opening, we'll start body-to-soul dialogs in our psyche with a comprehension of our place in the Universe and that we are the maker of our existence!

We will experience more prominent conditions of care, empowering us to imagine a superior life and make centered move to assist us with satisfying our latent capacity. We'll turn out to be exceptionally instinctive, have a decent memory, and we'll be able to comprehend with no issue.
Third Eye Guide – What is the Third Eye?

List of chapters

The third eye is our capacity to perceive what may be, to see potential.

Everybody approaches their third eye. For instance, when you suspect and follow up on it, you've utilized your third eye. Be that as it may, that is just the start. Your third eye is a sense, one you can create to be more refined and exact than simply being a hunch.

third eye

Dreams

Being A Seer

Instinct

Getting Visions

What is the Third Eye?

The third eye is established in the pineal organ. While the pineal organ may be the point of convergence for the intuition, the third eye is in reality significantly more than simply preparing yourself to interface with the pineal organ.

The Third Eye is a characteristic piece of each individual. One approach to consider it is as a "meta" organ that comprises of your brain and the entirety of your faculties cooperating as a bigger, all the more dominant tactile organ that the pineal organ at that point goes about as a point of convergence to make a dream. The Third Eye is a cunning piece of normal development that enables you to see the examples throughout your life. Significantly additionally stunning, your third eye can uncover these examples to you by overlaying this data over your different faculties.

As a sense, your third eye can be utilized from numerous points of view. Diviners utilize their third eye to comprehend shrouded associations and answer questions. Vitality laborers 'feel' the energies around them and to then deliberately control that vitality. What's more, every time you have compassion, you are utilizing your third eye to contact and feel the feelings of others. Numerous different models exist for how individuals utilize the Third Eye.

One outside asset to consider is this book: Third Eye: Third Eye, Mind Power, Intuition and Psychic Awareness: Spiritual Enlightenment

Seeing with the Third Eye

To see how the third eye functions, we should take a gander at how it is conceivable to utilize the Third Eye to detect and outwardly decipher vitality around us. It's conceivable to see Motion (for instance a vehicle moving), Activity (you driving the vehicle) and Exchange of Energy (consuming the gas). Include our ability of detecting and anticipating potential (having the option to foresee where the vehicle goes dependent on the streets and knowing the driver), as such observing where vitality, movement, and exercises will stream to after some time. Include this together into an inside visual guide, and you have quite recently extended how you see Energy playing out (the aftereffects of utilizing the vehicle/fuel/goal to drive you up the slope). By considering vitality to be a psychological overlay instead of only a unique idea, it turns into an unmistakable property of life that we can figure out how to detect and interface inside a more profound way.

BODY and LIGHT MEDITATION

Is it conceivable to truly 'see' vitality? Not straightforwardly. While our eyes can see the aftereffects of vitality in real life, seeing vitality legitimately is something else out and out. Our eyes just 'see' what they are intended to see, light. What our third eye does is process data and afterward overlay that data over our different faculties in such a manner we would then be able to translate and collaborate with vitality in an increasingly exact way. Thusly, we can comprehend where the vitality is, and we can 'see' it.

This bodes well, things being what they are. The psyche has made sense of something and needs to let us know. The simplest path for it to do this is to utilize what it as of now approaches: our five typical faculties.

Understanding the Third Eye
This brief general prologue to the third eye discusses:

(1) What is Potential?

(2) What is the Third Eye Physically?

(3) How does the Third Eye Manifest Itself?

(4) Is the Third Eye Something to Fear?

(5) More About Fear and the Third Eye.

(6) Am I Crazy?

(7) How to Express Your Third Eye Visions.

(8) Picking a Third Eye Practice and Community

(9) Learning How to Optimize Our Visions.

(10) Can You Manifest Real Things with the Third Eye?

(11) Can You Travel to Different Worlds with the Third eye?

(12) Can I Share What I See?

(13) How to Develop Your Skills in the Third Eye.

(14) An Example of Using the Third Eye

(15) Practice Interpreting Your Visions.

Individuals will cause the capacity to show up as a mysterious power having the option to "see" or "foresee" forms, occasions, possibilities which are not physically present. Be that as it may, it's an undeniable and substantial ability.

Since such a great amount of relies upon your capacity to translate results, there is a ton of space for mistranslation between the "realities" and what your third eye comes back to you. Likewise, in light of the fact that every one of us sees things in an unexpected way, it very well may be dangerous to share what we see with others. For instance, when we hear the word 'cup', every one of us may envision a totally extraordinary cup. What one individual will detect is not the same as another.

Obviously, shared traits exist. We are human and our structure, our inclination help push us towards regular baselines of experience. Be that as it may, the one of a kind sort of every individual additionally guarantees that every one of us sees the world from an alternate point.

It shouldn't be astounding, at that point, that there are such a large number of various otherworldly practices to investigate all the various view of the world we hold.

Consider an individual who sees atmospheres or light. Emanations are in truth such a data overlay. Your cerebrum can process visual data, however the picture it makes for you isn't constrained to what originates from your eyes. Think about what you see on this page as you read it. You aren't seeing dark lines. You are seeing words and afterward ideas and thoughts overlaid over them.

Presently imagine yourself taking a gander at someone else. You don't simply observe what the person in question is wearing. Your entire neural system, brain and sense organs structure a bigger increasingly delicate radio wire that gets on vitality and examples before you. There are such a large number of signs before you that educate you concerning the individual's enthusiastic state, prosperity, level of interruption, thus numerous different elements. Your third eye has a great deal to impart to you thus it places this data into what you see by including an emanation. As a general rule what you are seeing is marginally extraordinary over what's going on: however your brain is continually changing your experience to give you additional data to work with. In the event that you take a gander at the logical research you will find the brain is always altering our recognition. So the third eye utilizes this common mental ability to adjust our recognition to include additional information more than we understand.

Seeing qualitys, chakras or vitality can show up as a magical power, contingent on an individual's degree of ability. In any case, it is only that: an undeniable and unmistakable expertise, one that can be educated. An individual can even be instructed how to see emanations in a standard manner.

THIRD EYE MEDITATION

Individuals commit an error to believe that the third eye is a functioning procedure. Indeed, a typical inquiry is:

"What does the Third Eye DO?"

The third eye is a sense. Faculties do nothing straightforwardly other than hand-off data to you.

What do your eyes effectively do? Nothing, you can't shoot lasers or warmth vision from your eyes. Your eyes rather return visual data.

What does your hearing effectively do? Nothing, you don't intentionally make clamor out from your ears. Your ears rather return sound-related data.

The third eye is a sense. It returns data about possibilities and enthusiastic state. Possibilities speak to what may be, and Energetic state is about how something is being held.

The activity, or DO is the manner by which you utilize the data you gain from your faculties.

Such a large number of individuals in the event that they just tune in and, at that point followed up on what they heard, wouldn't stumble into so a lot of difficulty. Moreover in vision, such a significant number of individuals don't really "look" and botch chances as they surge past things.

The third eye is a sense, it returns data on what may be and furthermore lively states. With it you can detect someone else's feelings: that is sympathy. The third eye you can let you feel how an individual is getting along. It can give you how an individual's biography is streaming. With the third eye, you can get suspicions of what may be ahead, behind or far out.

Reflection and Perception

Grow Perception

Become Lucky

GUIDED MEDITATIONPERSPECTIVE

Your Third Eye Could Already Be Open.

Ordinarily the stunt isn't opening the third eye yet to remember we see more than we understand. For some individuals, it's as of now open (a great many people just squint through the third eye). The genuine issue is a great many people unwittingly disregard it through and through. For other people, it's something to fear such a large number of individuals effectively turn away when it is attempting to give you something.

Opening the third eye implies working on utilizing your intuition. The stunt is figuring out how to acknowledge it is there and afterward decipher what you are detecting over the long haul. The more serious issue is very numerous individuals power the procedure and afterward get overpowered by stories, yes stories! All the more strangely, the third eye is the main sense that gives us stories. We are human; to be human is to live with our accounts; we do have faculties to explore those accounts. The intuition is our prime sense we use to pursue a story and foresee where a story is going towards.

Since we use stories to make a guide of how to explore the world, Our psyche makes mental stories for us as dreams that the third eye works up to use as smaller than expected maps. To some extent to connect with the third eye is to turn into a storyteller, to see a story and afterward use it to help move all the more smoothly throughout everyday life.

Outrageous occasions like an emotional meltdown, injury, or other groundbreaking minutes can drive an individual's third eye open. Any circumstance that drastically changes an individual's encounter of the world can be the impetus for changing how they see potential.

The vast majority either don't tune in to their third eye, so they work somewhat harder to move through life.
Exercise Two:

Try not to make a dream greater than life. Very numerous individuals make a huge deal about a dream they experience. Be Calm!

Exercise Three:

Practice simply watching life stream around you. The third eye uncovers examples of the world unfurling around you. Thus, the more you comprehend the examples of nature, the simpler it is to comprehend what a dream can speak to.

We can spot Trends, and regularly our mind will sign us into a pattern with basic bits of knowledge and flashes of motivation. Such a significant number of third eye encounters can simply speak to a basic example unfurling. To constrain a dream to mean more than it wills divert individual from the basic example you just observed being uncovered.

So keep the elucidations as basic as would be prudent and afterward develop out extending the significance as you improve at deciphering your third eye encounters.

Exercise Four:

Back to Pause.

You stop while accepting an instinct. The third eye isn't utilizing the sensible thinking part about the brain. Subsequently, on the off chance that you start to think the minute you get a dream it disturbs the third eye process. So you delay to stop the remainder of your brain from demolishing the third eye minute.

Exercise Five:

The third eye is a wonderful sense; it grows how an individual associates with the world, adds another measurement to how we interface with everything. In any case, it's just one of numerous faculties. Individuals will in general center a lot just on one sense, and that confines an individual a lot at that point. So you must be patient and figure out how to utilize the entirety of the faculties together, or you are feeling the loss of the bigger world.

After you get a dream with the third eye you check all your different faculties, even utilize your rationale, you jab about and include different snippets of data to make a much increasingly complete picture if conceivable.

At the point when your different faculties return conflicting data, at that point you delayed down. Make sure to enable your instinct to reveal to you when to back off to delay and take a gander at everything around you. On the off chance that other data broadens and approves what you sense, at that point you push forward with more surety.

The third eye is a characteristic sense we as a whole have. The third eye is a sense to identify "what may be" or our feeling of potential. To open the third eye intends to additionally build up that sense to the point of staying alert and aware of the sense.

When the third eye is opened, it doesn't accompany an eyelid that we can simply close. It's increasingly similar to our ear, consistently on. The issue is this: a few people get overpowered by their faculties.

For instance, PTSD is a fantastic case of an illness for an individual excessively sharpened to data their faculties gives to them. A few people can be damaged by observing excessively!

Figuring out how to "close the third eye" is figuring out how to either deal with the third eye sense and how to disregard it indeed.

In the event that you need to close your third eye, at that point one methodology you can take is making your life ordinary, unsurprising and standard. Let's be honest current culture works admirably of closing individuals' vision of potential down. Individuals are excessively bustling attempting to expend others' vision.

Working with Your Senses

You can decide not to tune in.

For instance: since individuals can hear, doesn't mean a great many people tune in! In like manner you can instruct yourself to disregard your own dreams and your mind will simply adapt naturally avoid past the dreams.

On the off chance that you don't tune in to the third eye, the absence of utilization itself hoses down the third eye.

At long last:

Judgment is something contrary to potential, and it generally will close down the third eye.

On the off chance that you don't need the third eye: at that point judge it as being incomprehensible or converse with enough individuals who don't put stock in it. Confronting and tolerating others' judgment will rapidly restrict you and the third eye will leave rapidly accordingly.

Shutting the Third Eye

Craftsmanship by AaronMiller

THIRD EYE MEDITATION

BODY and LIGHT MEDITATION

The Third Eye and Energy Work

How would I utilize the third eye to work with vitality?

A short diagram is that you utilize the third eye in vitality work to see vitality. Anyway to change vitality is another arrangement of procedures. You can utilize breath, movement and other dynamic procedures to shape vitality. Qi Gong is ideal instances of this, where you use breath to work with your Chi/Qi or in Kundalini Yoga where you use reciting to work with Kundalini vitality.

There are numerous other dynamic methods to work and change vitality, however I will pressure that the third eye is the sense used to envision that vitality. We work with vitality with activities and our intuition encourages us control those activities.

Showing the Third Eye

Julie and I show others how to get to the third eye, yet know this capacity isn't hurried yet rather developed into after some time. Julie and I will show you how to develop quietly and completely into this expertise.

In the event that you are keen on adapting more the best spot to begin would be in an experiential way. We would either help you through a power creature recovery or by managing you on a shamanic venture. Every one of these encounters would be a way of legitimately utilizing the third eye to interface with the profound side of life. Soul speaks to the movement and associations with everything around us.

The most effective method to Open Your Third Eye And Awaken Your Psychic Gifts

Arousing your third eye opens your window to the otherworldly world. One approach to stir this is to take part in otherworldly practices, for example, contemplation.

The third eye, which is situated close to the pineal organ in your cerebrum, is essentially your window to the otherworldly world.

At the point when your third eye chakra is open, your physical and profound bodies are in finished congruity and you become considerably more associated with your instinct. Not exclusively will you trust in your premonitions more, however you'll likewise have the option to build up your clairvoyant blessings all the more effectively. Before long, you'll see that you can encounter sensations past your five "customary faculties."

An open and stirred third eye opens the entryway to incredible superconscious capacities just as a more clear, increasingly engaged, and adjusted condition of being. At the point when you're progressively associated with your profound self, you will access its interminable astuteness, so you'll additionally be significantly increasingly definitive and settle on better choices about your life.

Things being what they are, how would you start arousing your third eye?

Take part In Spiritual Practices Focused On The Third Eye

Contemplation, petition, and yoga, are the absolute most solid approaches to develop and enact your third eye. Envision your third eye, situated in the focal point of your brow, sparkling splendid purple and beating with all your breaths. As you take in and out, luxuriate in the light and vitality of your third eye and let yourself feel its brilliance all over your body.

These profound practices don't need to assume control over your life. Basically commit 10 to 20 minutes of your time ery day to ponder, ask, or practice yoga. Before long, your life will change and you will be glad for the changes, as you become more sensitive to your Higher Self and the otherworldly world.

Eat Good Food

Nourishment can assume a critical job in the prosperity of the chakras, since the physical and otherworldly bodies are intended to be in a state of harmony and associated. The nourishment that you eat influences your vitality, considerations, and emotions, so it's imperative to ensure that what you're placing into your body is unadulterated and solid.

Handled nourishment is neither unadulterated nor sound, so avoid eating a lot of these moment suppers for new foods grown from the ground, just as entire grains.

A few nourishments even explicitly bolster the third eye, especially dishes wealthy in iodine, for example, kelp, ocean growth, shrimp, lobster, kale, and bananas, among others. Cell reinforcements like crude cacao and apple juice vinegar will likewise assist flush with excursion destructive poisons and keep your body spotless and sound.

A lot of herbs are additionally known to invigorate the pineal organ, so devouring these will help on the off chance that you need to open your third eye. Hay sprouts and parsley are two that can be effectively added to your suppers, while home grown teas with rosemary, passionflower, and ginkgo biloba, are likewise extraordinary for this chakra.

It barely should be stated, yet make sure to drink bunches of water also, the best cell reinforcement around!

Support Yourself With Sunshine

The sun is a wellspring of intensity and vitality for every one of the seven chakras, yet it's especially steady of the third eye.

While it might be an impractical notion to gaze legitimately into the sun, light reflected from the retina is really known to actuate the pineal organ. In this way, when you're outside, discard the shades and let yourself appreciate the sun unobscured. Backhanded presentation to daylight is really essential for your two "standard" eyes, just as your third eye.

To help the enlivening of your third eye, get a decent portion of common light every day. Make it an ordinary piece of your daily practice, regardless of whether you lean toward getting your daylight by going for an early morning stroll to begin your day, taking your canine for a walk, or sitting at the recreation center for some reflection time toward the evening.

Not exclusively will you further the improvement of your third eye, yet investing energy under the sun gives you a solid portion of Vitamin D, which lifts the brain and soul, just as kicks melancholy. Simply remember to apply a layer of sunblock, particularly when you realize you will be under the sun for quite a while.

Figure out how To Work With Crystals And Oils

Precious stones and basic oils are significant apparatuses that animate the distinctive chakras, so when you are keen on arousing your third eye, you'll need to know which ones can assist you with doing as such.

Many purple precious stones sustains the third eye, including Amethyst, Purple Sapphire, and Purple Fluorite. Lapis Lazuli and Moonstone are additionally known to function admirably the third eye.

Figure out how to utilize these precious stones in a manner you're alright with, regardless of whether it's wearing them as adornments, conveying them in your pocket, laying down with them by your bedside table, or thinking with them routinely.

With regards to basic oils, a portion of the ones that actuate the third eye are sandalwood, franckincense, jasmine, patchouli, lavender, and rose, among others. It relies upon which oil you're utilizing, however basic oils are normally breathed in. Some incline toward saturating their bodies with them by utilizing body creams which contain these oils, while others place a couple of drops in a diffuser or nebulizer, so the entire room is injected with the fragrance.

Rehash Positive Affirmations And Mantras

Positive assertions, which are sure expressions or sentences, steer you away from the negative and assist you with concentrating on the energy that you need to show in your life. Keep in mind, what you think, feel, and accept, are what you show and turn into.

On the off chance that you need to open your third eye, you'll need to utilize confirmations that support your otherworldliness and feeling of direction, for example, "I believe my instinct and it will consistently lead me to the light," or "My third eye is unguarded with boundless intelligence and potential."

Reciting a mantra is very unique, in that mantras are only a solitary word or sound that contains ground-breaking otherworldly vitality. OM is the seed sound of the third eye, so have a go at rehashing it to yourself as you breathe out during reflection, supplication, or only a tranquil singular minute.

The most effective method to Activate Your Third Eye Using Meditation Techniques

The third eye is an otherworldly idea that alludes to an individual having the option to accomplish observation past common sight.

Otherwise called the 'inward eye', it is the entryway to internal domains and conditions of higher cognizance, past the physical world.

The third eye is usually connected with dreams, hyper vision, out-of-body-encounters (OBE), astral projection and the capacity to watch chakras and emanations.

Where is the Third Eye?

In Hinduism the third eye alludes to the temples chakra, situated around the center of the brow, marginally over the intersection of the eyebrows.

In Theosophy the third eye is said to be associated with the pineal organ, which keeps up light affectability and is answerable for the generation of DMT (dimethyltryptamine), a hallucinogenic medication which numerous mystics accept to be discharged in huge amounts at the snapshots of birth and passing.

It is said that through third eye contemplation, the third eye is initiated, DMT discharged and access to higher domains picked up.

The third eye is otherwise called the 6th chakra, and alluded to as "extrasensory sight", a word taken from the French language, signifying "clear vision" . This is fundamentally the 'intuition', which gives an individual the ability to get to data past the five physical faculties.

What Happens During Third Eye Meditation?

Third eye reflection opens up your extrasensory sight. Try not to stress in the event that you've never done this, since like eyes, everybody has a third eye; it simply needs initiating and preparing.

Opening the third eye permits a meditator to clear vitality squares and self-restrictions and discharges negative karma.

Individuals regularly find/get to new data and investigate more elevated levels of awareness during this type of reflection, and as referenced beforehand, this is likewise utilized as a pathway to astral projection and clear dreaming.

When you effectively initiate the third eye, beams of light will stream in and you will start to see striking hues, pictures, atmospheres and dreams. With training you will start to see all the more unmistakably, opening up pathways to more elevated levels of cognizance and otherworldliness.

In the event that you have extrasensory propensities they will start to thrive outside of your reflection. You may start to see the chakras and air energies of individuals, plants and creatures, and going ahead you may see other dimensional creatures and items.

Attempt this 21-Step Third Eye Meditation Technique

It is ideal to rehearse your third eye contemplation in the wake of having as of late woken up from a condition of rest; so best in the first part of the day or after an evening rest. The explanation behind this is the mind is as of now in a state helpful for contemplation, for example exceptionally loose in the theta state, with elevated internal mindfulness and instinct and low pressure/uneasiness levels.

It is additionally conceivable to enter third eye reflection as you are nodding off, be that as it may, this takes some training and it is ideal to begin the other path around first.

Most of astral explorers report distinctive, long scenes inside an hour of waking from rest, and in the early morning by and large.

Pursue these 21 stages:

Allot in any event 30-minutes for your reflection.

Mood killer your telephone and put forth a valiant effort to wipe out every single other interruption.

Ensure you're wearing happy with apparel.

Sit in the lotus position to guarantee your chakras are adjusted. In the event that you don't discover sitting leg over leg agreeable, at that point essentially rests.

Start by loosening up each muscle in your body, beginning with your toes and working as far as possible up to your head.

Envision each muscle, bone and tendon unwinding.

Presently move to a breathing reflection, as depicted here.

See the influx of quiet vitality come over your body. Feel its glow as it ascends through your body.

Easing back attract the vitality to the focal point of your head, in the middle of your eyebrows.

Try not to clutch any one however procedure or picture. Try not to make an effort not to think, simply let go of connections and repugnances as though nothing made a difference.

Feel yourself getting lighter and lighter, as gravity falls away.

Remain with your breath and picture a white bundle of light turning 360 degrees at the focal point of your brain.

See this ball extending and completely acknowledge its essence. Welcome to come into your possession.

As it extends let the light stream out through the focal point of your brow.

Once more, let go of considerations; simply let them rise and fall as they happen.

Give the light access and stay open to seeing whatever is put before you be it pictures, hues or data.

In case you're looking to interface with God (Mother Nature), or a soul manage, this is an ideal opportunity to get out and associate. This should be possible vocally (tranquilly and calmly) or inside.

Discuss your calling like a mantra until you get an indication of reaction. You'll know when it comes.

Do whatever it takes not to be frightened when it does; any stun or abrupt development may break the contemplation.

You may decide to approach your third eye for a message; for data or knowledge, or you may basically decide to simply be and take what originates from this edifying experience.

The experience may show up as dream-like, yet in time you will familairize yourself with the encounters and figure out how to develop and show higher information into your physical presence.

On the off chance that you solicited me a couple from years prior how to initiate your third eye I would have scrutinized your mental stability. However, as of late I delved into this subject due to my enthusiasm for supernatural quality, and I've discovered there's really a natural reason for the third eye. It exists and you can utilize it to facilitate your profound way.

Underneath you'll discover 15 best strategies for initiating it!

"Expelling a rock is now and again enough to change a predetermination."

— Samuel Sagan

What is the Third Eye?

It's really an organ in your cerebrum. Pineal Gland can even distinguish light getting through your "ordinary" eyes and control your rest cycle by discharging Melatonin into your framework. In numerous conventions it's been classified

The Eye is initiated by DMT, The Spirit Molecule, long contemplation, Kundalini experience, and numerous different strategies. It gives access to the universe of the obscure.

The third eye actuation crosswise over hundreds of years

The old Assyrians thought about it and delineated the Pineal as a secretive cone in their reliefs. The Egyptians demonstrated it through the Eye of Horus. Freemasons included it their rich imagery. Antique looks of Nepal talk about it. Cathars of Southern France thought about it. Also, even Buddha has this cracking third-eye-edification speck on his temple!

lady contacting her third eye

Opening the eye by rehearsing the correct propensities

During my reflective practices, I frequently feel a slight weight in my skull. I don't know whether this is a direct result of the synchronization of the sides of the equator or is there any third-eye business going on there. Be that as it may, I truly CAN feel it. I've discovered that you can trigger it through your conduct and great propensities for the brain and body.

So how would you actuate your third eye? Here are 15 top thoughts:

1. Ruminate for 20-30 minutes per day

One capacity of the third eye is to conscious you from the fantasy reality you for the most part involve at this moment. Reflection is an incredible method to do it. It causes you to take a gander at the world all the more obviously and know about your environment and mental state.

Build up a propensity for day by day reflection (regardless of whether for 20-30 minutes). You can undoubtedly become familiar with the nuts and bolts with books like The Relaxed Mind by Dza Kilung Rinpoche.

2. Expend Turmeric in each structure

Turmeric is an amazing zest. It lessens the irritation in your body, however it likewise retains supplements and scrub your blood. Some Indian masters put the turmeric glue on their brows asserting it clears the mind from neurotoxins and stirs the third-eye. Turmeric is as yet an extraordinary thing to attempt, regardless of whether as an enhancement or a tea.

Turmeric for Health: 100 Amazing and Unexpected Uses for Turmeric

Turmeric for Health: 100 Amazing and Unexpected Uses for Turmeric

Amazon Kindle Edition

Brandon, Britt (Author)

$9.99

Purchase now on Amazon

3. Drink separated water

One thing is without a doubt: most faucet water the world over contains heaps of fluorides which is viewed as a poison. There's even an intrigue about governments' association in "calcifying" our pineal organs.

Anyway, attempt to drink the most ideal and most clear water. You can do it by purchasing brands that don't contain fluoride or introduce a water channel in the kitchen.

4. Haritaki – the Herb of The Gurus

Haritaki has been utilized in India for centuries where it is known as the "Ruler of Herbs". Masters like Paramahamsa Nithyananda prescribe it as an enhancement opening the third eye, just as improving visual perception, expanding vitality, and guaranteeing simplicity of processing.

The West is gradually making up for lost time to the advantages of this astounding plant, which is presently effectively accessible on the web.

5. Eat for the most part foods grown from the ground

Arousing the pineal organ is tied in with cleaning your psyche and body so you can see measurements of reality inaccessible to an undeveloped spectator. During my 10-day contemplation retreat I haven't eaten any meat and I've seen that my mind was much more clear. You can have a similar encounter.

The best nourishments for the third eye initiation are:

Watercress

Pineapple

Coconut

Banana

Avocado

Parsley

6. Utilize a non-fluoride toothpaste

Most of less expensive toothpastes contain fluoride which is viewed as a poison. When brushing your teeth, you swallow modest quantities of toothpaste which can mess wellbeing up in the long haul.

Luckily now available, we have non-fluoride toothpaste which is absolutely protected to utilize and particularly prescribed for youngsters. Try not to let any frightful toothpaste to upset your third-eye!

7. Attempt to maintain a strategic distance from hot showers (or utilize a shower channel)

In the event that you scrub down, the pores in your body open and all the faucet water poisons are gradually consumed by your skin. Once more, this can "calcify" your pineal organ. You can fix it by introducing an ace shower channel in your washroom or simply quit scrubbing down.

As another option, cold showers are incredible for your wellbeing and spare you some time so check out them.

8. Eat Tamarind

Tamarind is a tree indigenous to tropical Africa yet it's really a staple of the Ayurvedic custom. The natural products, bark, and mash of tamarind have numerous therapeutic uses and will assist you with getting free of the abundance fluoride put away in your body.

9. Tune in to Third-Eye Awakening Binaural Beats
10. Eat well green powders

I need to state that veggie powders transformed me. Just by blending them in warm water or adding them to your smoothies, you can unfathomably improve your degree of mental and physical vitality. The ones I prescribe are Spirulina, Moringa, Wheatgrass, and Matcha. Utilizing them all the time is the following stage to the refinement of your body.

third eye realistic

11. Evade a lot of electric light and radiation

Following your common circadian cadence is important to stir the third eye. That implies you ought to for the most part wake up at dawn and rest a couple of hours after the dusk. Your body at that point realizes how to keep up a significant level of enthusiastic soundness. Assuming, be that as it may, you're stuck to your workstation, the TV screen or your cell phone, you can upset this regular progression of vitality (particularly in the event that you do it directly before resting).

12. Sungazing

The pineal organ can really detect photons that experience your outside eyes. That is the reason sun looking is such a ground-breaking approach to fill it with more vitality. In mysterious conventions, light is constantly associated with profound arousing. Holy people tend to shine, and during the

Kundalini experience, you're submerged in clear light. Do you see the association?

13. Take Iodine supplements

Dominant part of the populace is lacking in Iodine, which assists with decalcification and flushing fluoride from your framework. Just by enhancing yourself with items like Lugol's Solution, you can limitlessly speed up in which your body gets cleared from poisons. You can likewise get Iodine by eating kelp, cranberries, potatoes, and yogurt.

14. Practice Yoga

Yoga is one of the most seasoned physical and profound practices on the planet. By contemplating it you can discover about chakras which are the vitality focuses in your body. The Pineal organ is associated with the crown chakra which is initiated with rehearses like Pranayama, Vipassana, and Yoga, which is incredible for balancing out your "vitality winds" or what the Chinese call "Chi".

15. Invest energy in nature

It's essential to get some time away from the PCs and steady interruptions they bring. Getting several messages and advertisements for every day makes us so occupied and keeps us from seeing the more extensive the truth that is practically around the bend. By setting off to a backwoods or into the mountains you can reconnect with your actual being, and you ought to do it in any event once at regular intervals.

The Two Ways to Open the Third Eye

Sadhguru: The most huge part of Shiva is that he opened his third eye. He did numerous different things – he moved, he pondered, he wedded twice. All that is fine, yet it is simply because he opened his third eye that we recall him even today. Following a great many years, despite everything we bow down to him on the grounds that there is not a viable alternative for knowing. To know is to be free. What's more, there is no real way to know except if your recognition is improved past its present constraints.

Shiva is huge in light of the fact that he saw what most individuals neglected to see. What is inconspicuous for an enormous fragment of mankind turned into a typical piece of his vision. That is the thing that the third eye implies. Individuals state when Shiva opened his third eye, fire left it. This fire demonstrates that inside himself, he consumed everything that he thought made a difference to him. Inside himself, he turned into an oven that consumed everything that can be singed. And afterward, from each pore of his body, rather than sweat and blood, debris turned out. This is to show that he consumed each smidgen of numbness – everything that one accepts as evident. When this was done, the opening of the third eye couldn't be denied to him.

The Two Ways

There are two different ways of opening the third eye. One way is, within has become an all out vacuum so the entryway gets sucked in and needs to normally open. The entryway gets limp and falls internal in light of the fact that there is nothing. Shiva has consumed not just his idea, his feeling, his connections and assets – he has consumed his very being. There is an all out vacuum. So the entryway fell internal and opened.

Another method for opening the third eye is you contain everything inside. You don't discover any articulation for your idea, feeling or whatever else. You couldn't significantly express a word. You will see, on the off chance that you stay quiet for four days, on the fifth day you will all of a sudden vibe like singing. On the off chance that you don't have the foggiest idea how to sing, you will need to yell since you need to give up. In any case, on the off chance that you don't release anything, so much weight will develop that the entryway will get thumped open from inside. This is another way.

The Middle Path

Nonetheless, in the event that you are political, on the off chance that you trust in the center way, that implies you don't wish to go anyplace. Individuals who put stock in the center way are resolved not to go anyplace in their life. The center way is only your customary range of familiarity, neither. It implies you are a full-time bull-toilet. It doesn't make a difference where you go, you do your very own stuff – that is the center way. The center way is a method for not getting anyplace, and after some time figuring this doesn't go anyplace.

The center way is a method for not getting anyplace, and after some time figuring this doesn't go anyplace.

Suppose you were strolling in the city and you went over a major stone. There are just two approaches around it. One way, a tiger is snarling. The other way, a fire is consuming. On the off chance that you think the center way is the most ideal way and stroll into the stone, it will just give you great exercise for some time. You don't go anyplace.

In this way, it is possible that you become void and the sheer intensity of vacuum will open it, or you manufacture a weight in you and it will blast open – these are the two different ways. The principal way is a superior alternative in such a case that you open the entryway by building pressure, it might open up today and shut itself tomorrow. Or then again, before enough weight develops, something different may crack in you and you may flee. It is a great deal of torment not letting a solitary idea or feeling discover articulation, not expressing a solitary word, not discovering articulation to a solitary sentiment or thought that emerges in your psyche. It can make you burst! However, on the off chance that you do hold everything unblemished, the third eye will open.

THE THIRD EYE IN BIOLOGY

The pineal organ speaks to the third eye in science, which produces melatonin. Melatonin controls circadian rhythms and conceptive hormones. This makes the pineal an ace controller of time, influencing our rest designs as well as our sexual development. Melatonin additionally influences our pressure and capacity to adjust to an evolving world. This third eye enacts when presented to light, and has various organic capacities in controlling the biorhythms of the body. It works in agreement with the nerve center organ which coordinates the body's thirst, hunger, sexual want and the natural clock that decides our maturing procedure.

Essentialness OF THE THIRD EYE

Building up the third eye is the entryway to everything natural—clairvoyance, hyper vision, clear dreaming and astral travel. The figment of detachment among self and soul breaks down when the third eye association is developed. Mystical methods for being are associated with the third eye, for example, how to be wakeful inside the fantasy, to stroll among substances and outperform the constraints of humankind.

WHY YOU SHOULD AWAKEN YOUR THIRD EYE

A blocked third eye or ajna chakra is said to prompt perplexity, vulnerability, skepticism, envy and negativity. Through an open and dynamic third eye, the most elevated wellspring of ethereal vitality may enter. While the physical eyes see the physical world, the third eye sees the genuine Divine world — a brought together entire with an unflinching association with soul and Source. A rundown of the advantages and capacities that the third eye brings include: clearness, focus, perspicuity, euphoria, instinct, satisfaction, conclusiveness and understanding. The third eye has been connected to dreaming, nature of rest, upgraded creative mind and air seeing.

HOW DOES CALCIFICATION OCCUR?

The calcification of the pineal organ is normal if the third eye isn't being utilized or because of diets wealthy in fluoride and calcium. Calcification is the development of calcium phosphate precious stones in different pieces of the body. This procedure happens as a result of poisons in regular items, similar to fluoride, hormones and added substances, sugars and fake sugars.

Task: CELEBRATE THE THIRD EYE

Most creatures have pineal organs, regularly bigger than human pineal organs, that drive instinctual information. While your pineal organ might be dismissed and decalcified, praise that you without a doubt have a pineal organ. Start your enactment practice essentially by sending appreciation to your third eye for your intrinsic instinctive capacities and your association with nature through the circadian rhythms that the pineal organ administers.

Go through 10 minutes every day deliberately enacting your third eye through tuning forks, contemplation, reciting, petition, move or yoga.

tuning-fork

Snap to Order a Third Eye Tuning Fork

SIX WAYS TO AWAKEN THIRD EYE

Through decalcification and initiation, recover your Soul's way to euphoric rapture and association with Source:

Stay away from FLUORIDE — Pay close thoughtfulness regarding the water in your life: faucet water is a wellspring of fluoride, which adds to pineal organ calcification. Fluoridated toothpaste is another conspicuous wellspring of fluoride in current weight control plans, as are inorganic produce and fake beverages made with sullied water. Consider adding water channels to your sink and shower spigots.

SUPPLEMENT YOUR DIET — The rundown of enhancements that help and detoxify the third eye is long and incorporates crude cacao, goji berries, garlic, lemons, watermelon, bananas, nectar, coconut oil, hemp seeds, cilantro, ocean growth, nectar, chlorella, spirulina, blue green growth, crude apple juice vinegar, zeolite, ginseng, borax, Vitamin D3, bentonite mud and chlorophyll are for the most part fixings that helper cleansing of the pineal organ.

USE ESSENTIALS OILS — Many fundamental oils invigorate the pineal organ and encourage conditions of otherworldly mindfulness, including lavender, sandalwood, frankincense, parsley and pine. Basic oils might be breathed in legitimately, added to body oil, consumed in a diffuser and added to bathwater.

SUN GAZE — The sun is an incredible wellspring of intensity. Look delicately at the sun during the initial couple of moments of dawn and most recent couple of minutes of nightfall to help your pineal organ.

Ruminate AND CHANT — Meditation enacts the pineal organ through expectation: consider envisioning the decalcification of the pineal organ, as its hallowed nature is lit up and straightforwardly associated with source. Reciting causes the tetrahedron bone in the nose to resound, which causes incitement of the pineal organ. Considering reciting "Om," otherwise called the sound of the universe, multiple times every day.

Work together WITH CRYSTALS — Crystals are compelling partners in the journey to stir the third eye. Use gems and gemstones in the purple, indigo and violet shading palette. This shading palette serves to stir, balance, adjust and support the third eye. Attempt amethyst, purple sapphire, purple violet tourmaline, rhodonite and sodalite. Spot the precious stone or gemstone between and marginally over the forehead during reflection.

The power of the third eye opening is something that everyone can really learn and feel.

It gives you access to deeper knowledge. Today, there is a collective awakening that changes the limiting conditions of humanity. Unfortunately, the pineal gland is also prone to calcification due to processed foods and fluoride in water. However, this does not prevent the third eye opening and your pineal gland may still be sending signals from time to time.

It's time to understand if the signs you've noticed lately are related to the awakening of your third eye.

Here are the signs to look out for:

#1. You begin to think more deeply about what is to come.

Your old perception of things seems superficial and you realize that what you see is only a fraction of what really exists. As a result, you begin to increase your frequency and your state of consciousness begins to change.

#2. With the third eye opening, you can see the colors and the light of the day in a very different way.

All the senses are changed. Colors can be seen clearer. You can smell strange smells. You can also feel or hear things that "should not really exist". This almost psychotic experience applies to anyone who accidentally experiences the third eye opening.

#3. If you experience the third eye opening, you may feel a headache.

This is a pressure on your temples. It's also a sign that your pineal gland is developing energetically, so it's starting to channel your kundalini energy even more.

#4. Reality does not seem to be that real anymore with the third eye opening.

If the third eye accidentally opens, you may feel disconnected from the real world. You can have this strange feeling as if you live in a dream; as if everything was a lie and nothing else is important.

#5. With your third eye opening, you experience a large number of synchronizations and mirror numbers.

Once your third eye is open, you move into a higher state of consciousness. You will understand there are no coincidences and you begin to notice all the synchronicities that have occurred around you.

#6. Your third eye opening gives you the ability to literally see the unity of all things.

With your third eye opening, you have access to higher states of consciousness and, consequently, to other dimensions. There is no separation between you and the others, between the observer and the observed, the individual and the collective, the creator and the creation.

#7. You are increasingly asking about the purpose of your life with the third eye opening.

As your third eye awakens, you may feel more distinct, such as the negative energy of your job, relationship, possibly, the true intentions of some of your friends and even family members. It's a pretty normal transitional period of your awakening.

#8. You know more about what you eat with the third eye opening.
With your third eye opening, your sensitivity to toxicity increases and you now know that even foods are just energy and information. So you're only looking for food that really nourishes you.

#9. Another sign that your third eye is opening is when you have incredible and clear dreams.
The kind of dreams you never forget, because you feel that you can control them, and you can recognize your true infinite self. These dreams are extremely vivid and you will see them as a world of augmented reality.

#10. Clairaudience is an extrasensory ability that you could develop with your third eye opening.
You hear inaudible frequencies and hear the words that people never speak because you can tune in

and experience those special frequencies. This special ability is called clairaudience.

You can experience the third eye opening with these tips.
Practice meditation.
Instead of trying to control your thoughts and attitudes during the practice of meditation (like most people), just try to observe what your body and mind are doing.

Exercise and drink plenty of water.
That is pretty great! Drinking water also helps eliminate toxins from your body and hydrate your brain.

Avoid fluoridated water and even toothpaste.
Studies have shown that fluoride, the chemical in drinking water and toothpaste, is responsible for the calcification of the pineal gland.

Get out of your comfort zone and explore alternative ideas out there.

Closed third eyes thrive in narrow-mindedness. One of the best ways to open your mind is to always remain intellectually curious.

Restrict and cut processed foods as completely as possible.
You're going to benefit from a significant reduction in the consumption of animal meat due to the hormones it contains. If you'd like to stick to eating meat, ensure that it's as organic as possible.

Drink herbs to cleanse the third eye and then experience the third eye opening.
Herbs are an effective tool to help you recalibrate your very own third eye. Try the herbal teas that contain Gotu Kola.

Third eye opening with mindfulness!
The best way to anchor yourself in the present moment is an exercise known as mindfulness.

Flood your body with antioxidants.

Antioxidants detoxify and strengthen your body, which is ideal for learning to open your third eye.

Explore your basic beliefs.
Fundamental beliefs keep folks trapped in limited ways of thinking that keep the third eye closed. Learn to truly explore and solidify your basic beliefs.

Eat whole foods, vegetables, and fruits.
Your diet is important because it directly affects your hormones, energy and, therefore, feelings and thoughts.

With your third eye opening, you can capture thoughts that are not yours. You become an intuitive thinker. You have the ability to feel what people are thinking around you. This is a sign that you have activated your pineal gland.
The intensity of the third enlightening is something that everybody can truly learn and feel.

It gives you access to more profound information. Today, there is an aggregate arousing that changes the restricting states of mankind. Shockingly, the pineal organ is likewise inclined to calcification because of handled nourishments and fluoride in water. Be that as it may, this doesn't counteract the third educational and your pineal organ may even now be sending signals every once in a while.

It's an ideal opportunity to comprehend if the signs you've seen of late are identified with the enlivening of your third eye.

Here are the signs to pay special mind to:

#1. You start to ponder what is to come.

Your old impression of things appears to be shallow and you understand that what you see is just a small amount of what truly exists. Therefore, you start to build your recurrence and your condition of awareness starts to change.

#2. With the third educational, you can see the hues and the light of the day in an altogether different manner.

Every one of the faculties are changed. Hues can be seen more clear. You can smell unusual scents. You can likewise feel or hear things that "ought not so much exist". This practically crazy experience applies to any individual who unintentionally encounters the third educational.

#3. On the off chance that you experience the third enlightening, you may feel a migraine.

This is a weight on your sanctuaries. It's likewise a sign that your pineal organ is growing enthusiastically, so it's beginning to channel your kundalini vitality significantly more.

#4. Reality doesn't appear to be that genuine any longer with the third educational.

On the off chance that the third eye incidentally opens, you may feel disengaged from this present reality. You can have this unusual inclination as though you live in a fantasy; as though everything was a falsehood and nothing else is significant.

#5. With your third educational, you experience an enormous number of synchronizations and mirror numbers.

When your third eye is open, you move into a higher condition of cognizance. You will comprehend there are no fortuitous events and you start to see every one of the synchronicities that have happened around you.

#6. Your third educational enables you to truly observe the solidarity of all things.

With your third enlightening, you approach higher conditions of awareness and, subsequently, to different measurements. There is no detachment among you and the others, between the spectator and the watched, the individual and the group, the maker and the creation.

#7. You are progressively getting some information about the motivation behind your existence with the third educational.

As your third eye stirs, you may feel progressively unmistakable, for example, the negative vitality of your activity, relationship, potentially, the genuine aims of a portion of your companions and even relatives. It's a quite typical transitional time of your enlivening.

#8. You find out about what you eat with the third enlightening.

With your third educational, your affectability to poisonous quality increments and you currently realize that even nourishments are simply vitality and data. So you're searching for nourishment that truly supports you.

#9. Another sign that your third eye is opening is the point at which you have staggering and clear dreams.

The sort of dreams you always remember, in light of the fact that you feel that you can control them, and you can perceive your actual endless self. These fantasies are very distinctive and you will consider them to be a universe of enlarged reality.

#10. Clairaudience is an extrasensory capacity that you could create with your third enlightening.

You hear quiet frequencies and hear the words that individuals never express since you can tune in and experience those exceptional frequencies. This extraordinary capacity is called clairaudience.

You can encounter the third enlightening with these tips.

Practice contemplation.

Rather than attempting to control your considerations and mentalities during the act of contemplation (like a great many people), simply attempt to see what your body and psyche are doing.

Exercise and drink a lot of water.

That is quite extraordinary! Drinking water likewise wipes out poisons from your body and hydrate your mind.

Keep away from fluoridated water and even toothpaste.

Studies have indicated that fluoride, the concoction in drinking water and toothpaste, is answerable for the calcification of the pineal organ.

Escape your usual range of familiarity and investigate elective thoughts out there.

Shut third eyes flourish in extremism. Perhaps the most ideal approaches to open your psyche is to consistently remain mentally inquisitive.

Confine and cut handled nourishments as totally as could be allowed.

You're going to profit by a noteworthy decrease in the utilization of creature meat because of the hormones it contains. On the off chance that you'd prefer to adhere to eating meat, guarantee that it's as natural as could be allowed.

Drink herbs to purify the third eye and afterward experience the third enlightening.

Herbs are a compelling device to help you recalibrate your own one of a kind third eye. Attempt the home grown teas that contain Gotu Kola.

Third educational with care!

The most ideal approach to stay yourself right now is an activity known as care.

Flood your body with cancer prevention agents.

Cancer prevention agents detoxify and fortify your body, which is perfect for figuring out how to open your third eye.

Investigate your essential convictions.

Key convictions keep people caught in constrained perspectives that keep the third eye shut. Figure out how to genuinely investigate and harden your fundamental convictions.

Eat entire nourishments, vegetables, and organic products.

Your eating routine is significant in light of the fact that it straightforwardly influences your hormones, vitality and, in this manner, sentiments and musings.

With your third enlightening, you can catch musings that are not yours. You become an instinctive scholar. You can feel what individuals are thinking around you. This is an indication that you have enacted your pineal organ.
The most effective method to OPEN YOUR THIRD EYE and KNOW WHEN IT'S BLOCKED

When was the last time you had a feeling that you expected to check in with somebody, leave a space, or had a glimmer of knowledge and at the same time something appeared well and good? These little instinctive minutes are your third eye chakra at its best.

At the point when your third eye chakra is adjusted you don't just observe however you comprehend. That internal knowing can be felt all through your whole body, in each cell. Sounds pleasant, isn't that so?

In the event that your third eye chakra isn't adjusted you'll have an entire other arrangement of appearances that aren't exactly as ideal, which I'll diagram later.

The third eye chakra is situated in the focal point of your forehead bone. In Sanskrit, this chakra is called Ajna and makes an interpretation of "to direction" or "to see." It is answerable for your instinct, creative mind, and is your association with having a profound comprehension of the physical domain and the otherworldly domain.

Before I plunge into how to open your third eye, I need to give you a few hints for perceiving when it's blocked.

IS YOUR THIRD EYE CHAKRA BLOCKED?

Issue dozing or a sleeping disorder

Disarray or tension about choices you have to make

Visit cerebral pains

Absence of creative mind

Uncertain of how to manage your life

Poor memory

Feel dismantled to contemplate, be peacefully, and do therapeutic exercises

The most effective method to OPEN YOUR THIRD EYE CHAKRA

THIRD EYE MEDITATION

Contemplation is the quintessential strategy for taking advantage of the intensity of your third eye chakra. This can be as straightforward as sitting discreetly for 5 minutes every morning. At whatever point I escape my contemplation practice, I'm constantly stunned by the amount of a distinction 5 minutes of reflection influences my day. Look at this past blog entry for 8 Simple Ways to Be Here Now to assist you with bringing more care into your day.

Here's a reflection to attempt explicitly for adjusting and opening your third eye chakra:

Clear 5-20 minutes of continuous calm time for yourself;

Sit with folded legs on the floor or situated on a seat;

Fix your spine, lift your shoulders up and back and close your eyes;

With your eyes shut, point them both towards the focal point of your temples bone at your third eye chakra;

Concentrate on the breathe in and the breathe out of your breath;

With each breathe in envision a profound purple gleaming light growing around your third eye focus. As you breathe out it diminishes and afterward becomes greater and more brilliant with each breathe in.

When you subside into a cadence, rehash this mantra: I am associated with my higher self. I realize that I am constantly guided. I settle on choices easily and effortlessness. I acknowledge and trust the way I am on. My instinct is my guide. OM. (OM is the bija mantra for the third eye chakra, so don't hesitate to recite it more than once and truly coax it out!)

Rehash the mantra as frequently as you need.

When you're prepared to complete discharge your eyes, discharge any power over your breath, stop the mantra and rest for a couple of seconds.

Precious stones and SYMBOLS

The most intense gems for your third eye chakra are amethyst, lepidolite, celestite, and azurite.

Precious stone master, Judy Hall, clarifies the advantages of azurite, "Azurite guides mystic and instinctive improvement. It asks the spirit toward edification. It rinses and invigorates the third eye chakra and adjusts to profound direction."

Wear any of these gems or an image of the third eye as a token of your objective to remain associated with your instinct. We have structured an amethyst point gem ideal for associating with your third eye and an assortment of third eye propelled rings that you can shop here. You can likewise rest any of these stones on your third eye for included advantage.

Thinking about YOUR PINEAL GLAND

Physically, your third eye chakra legitimately identifies with your pineal organ. Your pineal organ is a modest, rice-sized organ tucked within your mind. It is a piece of your endocrine framework, it discharges melatonin and is liable for keeping up your circadian beat. Research done on the relationship among's reflection and the pineal organ have demonstrated expanded action and melatonin creation in the pineal organ during contemplation.

There are numerous nourishments and ecological elements that can influence it both adversely and decidedly. Fluoride can negatively affect your pineal organ. Abundance fluoride can develop in your pineal organ and cause it to become calcified, reducing the viability of your third eye.

To think about your pineal organ, attempt to remove fluoride of your eating routine as much as you can. Here are a few nourishments that can help in expelling abundance fluoride from your body and help decalcify your pineal organ:

Eat more iodine rich nourishments like broccoli, spinach, and ocean growth. Iodine rich nourishments are useful for some reasons yet can likewise help purge fluoride from your body.

Include increasingly crude apple juice vinegar to your eating regimen, in serving of mixed greens dressings or just in a blend of water and nectar. Crude apple juice vinegar has a high substance of malic corrosive which is useful for detoxifying the entire body.

Have some chamomile tea. Chamomile is a quieting tea that can help alleviate an overactive pineal organ.

Murkiness and LIGHT (MAYBE)

Take a stab at limiting light contamination in your room around evening time. Your pineal organ controls your circadian musicality so it tends to be gainful to give yourself time in the genuine dull. Give closing a shot all light from the outside, and any inside lights to give you some pre-rest time in a light free space.

On the other hand, some old convictions (that are as yet drilled today) recommend sun-looking to animate your pineal organ and third eye chakra. I don't generally feel good guiding you to go gaze at the sun since I've never attempted this and am not so much sure that I feel great doing it either! There's parcels to find out about it however, so in case you're keen on it I propose doing your own exploration on it.

7 Ways to actuate your third Eye Chakra

third Eye or Ajna Chakra is the sixth Chakra symbolized by 2 Lotus Petals. Hakini Shakti lives there and when you conjure Hakini Shakti, clear experiences, dreams and messages stream to you effectively and easily.

7 Ways to enact your third Eye Chakra

Mantras and Chanting

Mantra is a hallowed articulation, sound, a syllable, word or gathering of words in Sanskrit accepted by specialists to have mental and profound forces. Mantras are incredible and it works better on the off chance that it is recited multiple times ordinarily for in any event 40 days. I have had astonishing outcomes with different Mantras! Here are 3 Powerful Mantras for opening your third Eye Chakra.

Reciting these Mantras(just pick 1 from these 3) 108 times regularly for an all-encompassing timeframe will open and lift your third Eye Chakra. You may feel unsteady at first, experience migraines or weight on the third Eye zone when you start reciting these Mantras. I have just actuated your third Eye Chakra so you probably won't encounter any of these.

Om-Om is the seed sound of the sixth Chakra(Ajna or third Eye Chakra). Simply reciting Om a few times each day will initiate your Ajna Chakra.

Om agya-chakraa-bahja-nilayāyei namaha-This is the Mantra of Goddess Lalita Tripura Sundari who sits on the third Eye as Hakini Shakti (who leads the Ajna Chakra).

I prescribe you start reciting these Mantras on a New Moon or whenever during the Waxing watery Moon (which means Moon must get greater in one of the Water Signs, ideally Cancer or Pisces).

You will feel the distinction very quickly! You can keep a check utilizing your fingers or Japa (Mala Beads) that accompanies 108 dabs to assist you with keeping a tally of your Mantra.

Pressure point massage Tapping

Probably the most straightforward approaches to keep your third Eye Chakra solid and dynamic is by applying pressure on your third Eye. Pressure point massage point GV 24.5 which is directly in the center of your temples is an Acupressure point for invigorating your third Eye Chakra. Tenderly tap or press that region for around 2-3 minutes regular. You can even back rub that region in a roundabout movement for a couple of moments ordinary. Far and away superior is utilizing any third Eye Chakra Oil and afterward utilizing Acupressure or Massage.

Bindi

Have you at any point seen Hindu ladies wearing tattoo/bindi/speck on their third eye Chakra? Bindi is worn precisely on the GV 24.5 point! Stunning right? Did you realize that it originates from a conviction that if a lady wears a bindi/tattoo on her third Eye Chakra it causes her interface with the celestial female side effectively and furthermore shields her third Eye Chakra from any Psychic assault? Bodes well right? You don't need to utilize Bindi in the event that you are not feeling guided to. I have by and by seen a colossal contrast when I wear a Bindi and when I don't. It unquestionably makes me feel increasingly ladylike so it really enacts my Sacral Chakra as well! It additionally makes me feel less depleted when I am around antagonistic individuals and my instinct is at top when I wear Bindi. You can sport indigo or purple Bindi during your reflection or recuperating work to help your instinct.

Shading Therapy (Chromotherapy)

Shading is my preferred apparatus to translate divine messages! I can't envision an existence without dynamic hues! Think about those hallucinogenic splash-color enchantment! Truly, as a Hippie on the most fundamental level I love to work with hues!

Shading treatment can do ponders for enacting your Chakras!

There are 4 different ways to utilize Colors to initiate your third Eye Chakra.

Warrior Goddess Training

Indigo or Purple Foods

Homeopathic Color Remedy

Indigo or Purple Light

Indigo or Purple Foods

You can eat indigo or purple shaded nourishments to enact the third Eye Chakra. Blueberries, Figs, Raisins, Blackberries, Prunes, Plums, Eggplant, Purple Cabbage and so forth. Savor water Indigo or Purple shaded Bottle and feel the distinction.

5. Shaded Toning

Indigo or Purple Light

Shaded light treatment otherwise called hued conditioning is a phenomenal method to open your third Eye Chakra! You can purchase a shaded light treatment gadget and use on your third Eye Chakra. You can likewise utilize zero watt shaded bulb, switch it on and sit in the space for at some point to retain the vitality.

Purple Glasses–Another route is to wear an excellent Indigo or Purple shaded glasses for 10-15 minutes regular. It is much increasingly incredible on the grounds that Eye is related with the third Eye Chakra!

Precious stone Therapy

You can utilize Lapis Lazuli, Sodalite, Amethyst, Selenite, Moonstone, Azurite, Dumortierite, Celestite or Angelite to actuate your third Eye Chakra. Apophyllite with Stilllbite, Lemurian Quartz, Herkimer Diamond are other scarcely any gems that can enact your third Eye and Crown Chakra.

There are a few different ways to utilize these Crystals. You can wear them as adornments, convey it in your pocket or spot it under your cushion. Setting one of the gems under your pad is significantly progressively incredible in light of the fact that the third Eye Chakra is related with dreams and dreams.

You can work with any of the above recorded stones. Trust your instinct when choosing any precious stone. Once in a while gems will discover you so simply be available to getting the messages from the Universe.

You can likewise tie a bit of third Eye precious stone pendulum or directed crude stone toward something like an adornments holder or anything where you can hang the gem tied string. Presently rests directly beneath the gem ensuring that the precious stone is indicating your temples zone. Sit for 10-15 minutes with eyes shut. Picture indigo or purple light flooding your third Eye Chakra and clearing every one of the blockages with it's lively light.

You can likewise utilize a little Pyramid made of one of these stones to clear the blockages. Simply rests, place a pyramid on your third Eye and imagine your preferred third Eye image like Om, Purple/Indigo shading light, your Spirit creature associated with the Third Eye like Peacock, Eagle, Hawk and so on. You can likewise imagine a lovely lotus blossom sprouting gradually unfurling your clairvoyant blessings. Special insight for clear observing, Clairsentient for clear feeling, Claircognizant for clear knowing and Clearaudience for clear hearing. Whatever blessing that you need to stir center around that feeling.

6. Breathing strategy

Pineal Gland Cleansing

Pineal Gland is the endocrine organ related with the Ajna Chakra. So center around keeping this organ solid by diminishing synthetic compounds and poisons in your nourishment and condition. Something else that hinders this organ is Fluoride. Fluoride is neurotoxin so it gradually harms your sensory system which will naturally obstruct your third Eye Chakra.

Maintain a strategic distance from fluoridated toothpaste. Go for a characteristic one like Earthpaste or whatever other brand that doesn't utilize fluoride.

Heavenly Basil imbued water is fantastic for fluoride detox! Simply put some crisp or dried Basil in your water bottle or injecter and drink it day by day. You can likewise include crisp lemon cuts, cucumber or mint to make it all the more energizing. Basil likewise helps your insusceptibility keeping your respiratory framework solid.

Another nourishment that help with fluoride detox is Tamarind.

In the event that you feel too bleary eyed after your third Eye Chakra begins to open at that point remember to ground your vitality every now and again.

Have you at any point heard the articulation, 'Be cautious what you wish for'? For certain individuals, the opening of the third eye can give them things that they truly would not like to see. For other people, it's a voyage of edification. On the off chance that you are certain this is something you need to do, at that point please read on.

As indicated by wiki, the third eye (otherwise called the inward eye) is a magical and elusive idea alluding to a theoretical undetectable eye which gives observation past normal sight. In certain dharmic profound customs, for example, Hinduism, the third eye alludes to the ajna, or forehead, chakra. The third eye is alluded to the door that leads inside to inward domains and spaces of higher awareness. In New Age otherworldliness, the third eye regularly symbolizes a condition of illumination or the inspiration of mental pictures having profoundly close to home profound or mental noteworthiness. The third eye is regularly connected with strict dreams, hyper vision, the capacity to watch chakras and airs, precognition, and out-of-body encounters. Individuals who are professed to have the ability to use their third eyes are in some cases known as soothsayers.

On the Above Top Secret site, an individual by the name of "pellian" expressed the accompanying:

I found an undeniable method that will build your profound recognition by a thousand crease. I won't tell anyone what it is or where I learned it since Some may pull in exceptionally abhorrent substances and conceivably devastate themselves over it.

The absolute first night I attempted this I had an altogether different sort of dream which I had not had previously. The substance doesn't mean anything other than I deviate.

The day after I notice that occasionally my mindfulness would move and my vision appears to be changed for a minute. I imagined this is truly cool. I do the activities again before long. same thing around evening time. I see hues and shapes that pursue my vision. These were there on the off chance that I shut my eye in complete haziness or opened them in the extremely diminish light of my room. These appeared to be objects or some likeness thereof that emitted a diminish shine and had a woven example.

As I rehearsed it sounds extremely insane however I imagine that these activities made a type of vitality that pull in astral structures. One night, I woke up and saw this thick rope hung from my window ledge to the entryway. Right now I comprehended what it was. I tragically touched this creature or thing and felt a shock like power. I was unquestionably alert I promptly felt debilitated and had cools all over my body.

I proceeded with the activities two weeks after the fact. I was truly near rest and a blue ring of light that vacillated like a butterfly came into my room. I turned on the light and the ring persevered of about a second after and I again felt a sting I my side and similar chills. I guarantee that I am not dreaming and completely conscious.

On the off chance that this isn't some insane visualization, at that point whatever I have been doing is either illuminating me like a patio light to pull in moths or these substances are coming through to this world by means of my awareness. A pipedream can't influence you physiologically to make a stun impact.

I likewise have seen that when did the activities something appears to emerge in my room.

The degree of discernment was mind blowing. Be that as it may, was not worth being troubled by these elements.

Chapter four Advantages of third eye awakening

Our regular daily existence and the advanced style of being rationally occupied can prompt us putting some distance between our natural endowments. Here we investigate the 6 of the most mainstream focal points that accompany initiating the Brow Chakra.

Peruse: Activate Your Natural Relaxation Response In 7 Minutes

1. More noteworthy Awareness

The powerful arousing of your 6th chakra opens our eyes from otherworldly laziness.

This enables us to start to see "Reality" that encompasses us.

This means you start to see the world all the more obviously.

You will most likely feel a longing for opportunity and to live in a world loaded up with adoration, empathy and truth.

Inevitably, you will feel and see the interconnectedness with everything around you in nature and build up a solid bond with the Universe.

This is a profound sense that enables you to see the magnificence no matter what and to understand that your physical I isn't your actual nature.

2. Mystic Powers/Empathy.

Your senses are as a balanced compass that focuses you in the "right" bearing to accomplish what your spirit is searching for.

At the point when the Ajna awakens, you can peruse instinctual flag far simpler until they become practically like another sense, subsequently the term intuition is gotten from.

It's practically similar to you recognize what will occur and what will be the consequences of specific occasions.

That is the reason a few people believe that the most eminent prophets within recent memory had an open third eye constantly.

The inclination that we are all piece of a similar entire additionally turns out to be clear and you are equipped for sympathy with others, realizing that they are a piece of a similar all inclusive awareness.

3. Laws of Attraction/Space Order.

Because of enlivening the Muddy Pellet (another name of the third eye), the Brow chakra is initiated, which thusly encourages to adjust your seven chakra framework.

At the point when you are stimulated and in amicability with the Universe, you resemble a monster magnet for occasions, individuals, circumstances and so on.

By outfitting the intensity of the positive plan, appreciation and love, you can show substantially more excellence in your life.

You will become mindful that the quantity of valuable "incidents" will extraordinarily increment.

4. Clear Dreams/Lucid Dreaming.

Since your pineal organ directs your rest cycles, you will find that you rest much better and that your fantasies are progressively distinctive.

You could likewise be clear dreaming.

This implies you will feel that you can control your fantasies and you will have the option to understand your actual interminable self and the unending potential outcomes that exist in a condition of rest.

Also, you will understand that this universe of dreams is equivalent to "this present reality" wherein we live. For instance, the way that we have boundless potential outcomes and we are generally bosses of our own universe.

5. Astral Travel/Astral Projection.

At the point when the third eye interfaces with this degree of presence where there is no reality, our spirit can transcend the physical body and astral travel in existence.

Astral projection is one of the advantages accompanying the enactment of your third eye.

It can go anyplace known to man and whenever known to mankind.

Numerous individuals belive that when we dream, we really astral travel, and with wide opened third eye we can deliberately astral travel while we are wakeful, for instance, when we are in a condition of reflection.

6. Creative mind/Creativity.

With actuated pineal organ, you are consistently associated with the plane of presence where our spirits live.

In the plane of presence, there is no time or space, only an interminable love and truth – everything that has occurred and will ever happen as of now exists in the plane of presence.

Opening your third eye chakra.

In the wake of associating with it, you will find that your creative mind and imagination are too charged.

You gain the capacity to discover brisk answers for issues much effectively on the grounds that every one of the answers for every conceivable issue on the planet exist in the higher planes of consciousnes.

Alongside the capacity to have clear dreams and clear dreaming, your creative mind will be shimmered to an unheard of level.
Sustaining and Nourishing Your Pineal Gland To Open Your Third Eye

The pineal organ, so named on the grounds that its shape looks like a pine cone, sits just between the privilege and left halves of the globe of the mind and is liable for creating various synapses, for example, melatonin and serotonin. Be that as it may, numerous spiritualists and old societies have alluded to the pineal organ as the "third eye."

The pineal organ is known as the third eye in light of current circumstances. Analysts have found that the pineal organ, similar to our eyes, contains photoreceptors and is even enacted by the light that gets through our eyes. It reacts to light by creating serotonin and to obscurity by delivering melatonin that initiates rest. Furthermore, when daylight is transmitted to the pineal organ, this daylight can assist break with bringing down a portion of the unsafe synthetic concoctions that may encrust the pineal organ. It is the development of these synthetics that is accepted by spiritualists to keep the pineal organ from working as it should.

The most effective method to Detoxify and Decalcify Your Pineal Gland

Your pineal organ isn't secured by the blood-mind hindrance, which implies that it has no additional guard against poisons that may enter your circulation system. Manufactured calcium and engineered fluoride, specifically, appear to unfavorably influence the pineal organ, debilitating its capacity to process photons of light and produce synapses. Note that the worry is manufactured calcium and fluoride, not supplements that normally happen in vegetables, for instance.

To start to completely enact your third eye, at that point, you should initially freed the pineal organ of these poisonous synthetic compounds that keep it from working accurately. You can start to do this by drinking cleaned water and suspending any nutrients, supplements, invigorated nourishments, and toothpastes that contain manufactured fluoride and calcium.

Nourishment for Your Pineal Gland

Notwithstanding detoxifying your pineal organ, you ought to consider likewise how to effectively sustain your pineal organ with your dietary decisions. This can bolster a definitive opening of your third eye.

To start, you ought to be aware of eating natural plants and creature items. Some would suggest that you seek after a vegetarian diet just, maintaining a strategic distance from every single creature item.

There are explicit nourishments accepted to invigorate the pineal organ. These include:

Apple juice vinegar (unpasteurized)

Beets

Cacao beans

Grass juices

Green vegetables

Reishi mushroom tea

Turmeric

Step by step instructions to Activate Your Pineal Gland

A decent spot to start in you need to progress in the direction of enlivening your pineal organ is to with customary reflection. Contemplation is useful for both the body and the psyche yet in addition for our chakra framework. In particular, contemplation enables you to encounter more prominent conditions of clearness and instinct. Unquestionably, joining a steady otherworldly network, for example, The Way International, can be useful too.

In the wake of rehearsing reflection normally for quite a while, you might be prepared to move towards the further developed act of Kundalini Yoga. Kundalini practice attempts to initiate your chakras. In particular, it attempts to stir Kundalini vitality, which rests at the base of the spine. This vitality can move upwards through the spine and to the pineal organ, further opening the third eye.

A few specialists accept that Ayahuasca can be utilized to open the third eye. Ayahuasca is produced using the Ayahuasca plant local to parts of Central and South America. Ayahuasca is an incredible laxative that may purify the body from an assortment of poisons, including those that restrain the pineal organ. Also, Ayahuasca can make the compound DMT, or di-methyl-tryptamine, bio-accessible, prompting a characteristic opening of the third eye chakra.

Customary fasting is additionally prescribed by some as an approach to stir the pineal organ and open the third eye. Indeed, even a 24-hour quick can expand detoxification normally and increment the generation of Human Growth Hormone, which invigorates the creation of new synapses. It ought to be noticed that while fasting, you should drink a lot of decontaminated water.

What Are the Benefits of Opening the Third Eye through the Pineal Gland?

Having a sound, clear third eye offers numerous advantages, both otherworldly and functional. These include:

More noteworthy mindfulness—you will start to comprehend reality with regards to your general surroundings and will understand that "you" are not your physical self.

More noteworthy compassion—you are probably going to turn out to be progressively empathic, not simply sympathetic. That is, you will be intently sensitive to the passionate states and even contemplations of others.

More noteworthy instinct—you are probably going to start to just know things that you have no consistent method for knowing. You may know the result of specific occasions before they occur.

Increasingly striking dreams/clear dreaming—on the grounds that your pineal organ manages your rest cycle, your fantasy state is probably going to be influenced by an opening of the third eye. You may discover you have dreams that are practically prophetic in nature or that give you understanding. 7 Life Changing Benefits Of Opening The Third Eye

What is the third eye?

The third eye chakra, otherwise called anja chakra in Sanskrit, situates the eye of the spirit. A completely actuated third eye enables you to see the world through a higher point of view. Envision having the option to see enthusiastic structures through the five detects. To feel vitality, see it and even hear its vibration. Mystic recognition is just conceivable with a stirred third eye.

The third eye is a nerve group connected to the pre frontal flaps of the mind that impact and influence clairvoyant discernment. The pineal organ is at the focal point of this nerve group and when enacted, awards the five detects the capacity to see vitality. This initiation is conceivable through the development and incitement of the third eye chakra.

For centuries, elusive schools and different religions viewed the pineal organ as the interfacing join between the physical and profound domain. However, it would take starts of these puzzle schools months/long stretches of exhausting preparing to enact the pineal organ.

In this quick moving present day age, you can really actuate it in merely weeks by reliably tuning in to this enthusiastically customized sound.

For what reason is the third eye chakra shut in any case?

All things considered, the third eye chakra isn't shut, simply under-working. Truth be told you would encounter serious issues if any chakras were shut, they work with the body and organs and assume a significant job in keeping up life by accurately appropriating/sifting/evolving vitality.

It is underworking because of different reasons, for example, preset molding of the psyche, vitality blockages, negative vitality, restricting convictions, and the calcification of the pineal organ.

The collection of fluoride in the pineal organ makes it solidify which makes it produce less melatonin, upsets its wake-rest guideline and ends its capacity to empower mystic discernment.

In this way, it is basic to clear your third eye chakra of blockages and decalcify your pineal organ in the event that you intend to stir your third eye. On the off chance that you power your third eye to stir rashly, you are probably going to draw in negative elements and become truly helpless against mystic assaults.

The vivacious programming in this ground-breaking sound field will in reality clear your third eye everything being equal and decalcify the pineal organ. Simultaneously, it will invigorate and develop the third eye open such that you experience all the positive advantages you see beneath.

Presently, everybody encounters various advantages after opening the third eye yet these are the advantages you can expect after opening it and building up your capacities through training.

7 Benefits of opening the third eye

1. More elevated level of cognizance free from pressure, tension or stress

An open third eye chakra will expand the vibration of your considerations and higher vibrational reasoning is fixated on the present minute. Uneasiness and stress is fixated on the future and stress is focused on the past. The chains of uneasiness and stress will never again drag you down and you'll rather encounter the rapture of being right now.

2. Stir your higher instinct

Opening the third eye resembles revealing another layer of reality you didn't know was there. You have most likely heard that you would have the option to see astral substances and airs however will you likewise comprehend what these elements convey and what these atmospheres state about somebody?

Yes.Eyes of the Universe, dynamic ecological foundations

The third eye chakra is likewise the seat of the instinct and awards you access to a more significant level of comprehension. Everything is basically known to your soul and a stirred third eye connects the association between your soul and your cognizant personality.

Allowed this more significant level of comprehension, you will start to acknowledge how we are altogether associated and a piece of an all inclusive cognizance. Your instinct will uncover the reasons why certain occasions throughout your life occurred and how you turned into the individual you are today. Be that as it may, above all, you will...

3. Be coordinated to your actual way

With direct access to your instinct, you will know precisely what you have to do as of now to advance throughout everyday life. Even better, you will be in your spirit's course and coordinated onto the way that will present to you the most satisfaction.

No more disarray. Not any more scanning for answers. They are all inside as they generally have been. Be that as it may, presently you will realize how to discover them.

4. Tap into your concealed mystic capacities and acquire dangerously sharp senses

The entirety of history and everything that will occur later on has occurred right now. Everything is here at this point. Our third eye chakra rises above space/time and is sensitive to this reality. This is the reason clairvoyants (with open third eyes) are regularly ready to determine what will occur later on. What's to come is natural information that can be taken advantage of with the third eye chakra.

Sense threat drawing closer. Know the correct answer. Make the best decision. That is the thing that an uplifted instinct will result in.

You will likewise have the option to see individuals' qualitys and astral substances that abide around. As I referenced, you strip away a layer of the real world and perceive the truth about it. We are enthusiastic creatures and are altogether interconnected. Our considerations show in the astral. These are a portion of the things you will start to comprehend and encounter for yourself with an open third eye.

5. Outfit the intensity of the law of fascination and show the existence you want

Higher vibrational contemplations apply more power and show considerably more rapidly. You will start to see numerous synchronicities with an open third eye chakra as your musings often show into 'incidents'.

This degree of thought is focused on the present minute and the present is the wellspring of all the vitality known to man.

In the event that you have ever attempted to show your wants by envisioning you have it, you may have fizzled on the grounds that your creative mind was dominated by your uneasiness to acquire what you wanted and worry of not having it. Indeed, you might not have even had the option to unmistakably picture what you needed.

You can expect a substantially more striking creative mind that is fixated on the present minute with an open third eye lastly exploit the law of fascination.

6. Stir your virtuous creative mind and appreciate unlimited degrees of inventiveness

For the most part, individuals with dynamic third eye chakras (not really completely open) can envision obviously and have an incredible creative mind. This is on the grounds that the third eye can see into the astral domain and our contemplations are showed in the astral. An open third eye awards you supreme clearness with your creative mind and empowers you to encounter your considerations as you did as a youngster.

With your cognizant personality more in line with the astral, it is more on top of the unlimited conceivable outcomes of the real world. Interfacing with the wellspring of creation actuates the creative mind.

7. Addition the capacity to clear dream and astral travel

The third eye enables you to deliberately witness the astral when you see substances, atmospheres or in any event, when you distinctively observe what you envision. It will likewise allow you the capacity to deliberately visit the astral domain in your etheric body.

A stirred third eye brings about a more significant level of mindfulness that goes past the egoic mind that is connected to the body. Attention to your vitality body can keep you conscious in any event, when your body nods off and enable you to enter the astral as your astral self.

This degree of mindfulness frequently enables you to stay cognizant in your fantasies too.

Numerous spiritualists have looked for pineal organ opening or third educational for quite a long time. There are various approaches to get to this state, and it is positively worth the exertion. Furthermore, the opening of your third eye will enable you to see the world, your place in it, and everyone around you with more prominent clearness and truth.

7 LIFE-CHANGING BENEFITS OF OPENING YOUR THIRD EYE

The idea of the third eye is one that many individuals are passingly acquainted with. Associated with the ajna chakra (the one situated in the forehead), this is the 6th chakra in the Hindu convention. While your two typical eyes enable you to see the physical world surrounding you, the third eye is related with instinct, the future, and in certain customs with the soul world also. While everybody has a third eye, not every person has set aside the effort to open it, and to see the world through it. The individuals who invest the energy and exertion to open this chakra, however, will find that doing so offers them various advantages in their everyday lives.

Advantage #1: IT BRINGS BALANCE TO YOUR OTHER CHAKRAS

Since the 6th chakra remains at the most elevated spot in the body, and is associated with what may seemingly be our most significant organ, it holds an uncommon spot of intensity and position. On the off chance that one can open up their third eye, at that point it will in general bring their different chakras into closer arrangement. This enables you to get a hold of yourself, making an inside congruity that lets you face the world as a brought together entire, instead of as somebody who is out-of-step with their own self as indicated by Psychic Gurus.

Advantage #2: YOU WILL GET BETTER SLEEP

At the point when your energies are not in arrangement, it can upset your rest similarly as most likely as though there was an excessive amount of weight on your hips, or something pushing into your back. Since the ajna chakra is related with the cerebrum, and all the more critically with the pineal organ, it has a lot of impact over your rest examples and quality. Notwithstanding guaranteeing you show signs of improvement nature of rest, however, opening your third eye will likewise enable you to all the more plainly observe your fantasies, as they are most effectively deciphered through the perspective of this specific chakra.

Advantage #3: YOUR CREATIVE ENERGIES WILL FLOW

The third eye is related with seeing things outside yourself, yet it is likewise about observing into yourself, and the world that lives inside your psyche. By reinforcing and opening this chakra, you will have the option to connect with your inward innovativeness in manners that may have been troublesome or sporadic previously. The creative mind moves through this chakra, and keeping it open will enable you to take advantage of that piece of yourself without any difficulty than you've at any point experienced previously.

Consecrated Geometry Clothing

Advantage #4: PEOPLE WILL BE DRAWN TO YOU

While there are advantages to being in line with yourself, when you adjust your chakras, this likewise aligns you with the progression of the general energies surrounding you. You become some portion of the stream, instead of the stones attempting to separate that stream. As per Inner Outer Peace, this will cause individuals (and even occasions) to stream toward you. It resembles opening your third eye transforms you into a magnet; others will be attracted to it, regardless of whether they may not exactly get why, themselves.

Advantage #5: CLARITY AND FOCUS

We've all had those occasions where we understand worried about something. Possibly it was those bills we had coming that we didn't know we could cover, a discussion with a friend or family member about a troublesome subject, or simply broad disappointments with your work, your neighbors, or some other part of your life. All that pressure can burden you, however more significantly, it can cloud your brain and make it hard for you to see the arrangements that are directly before you. In the event that you open your third eye, however, it penetrates through the mist of pressure and disappointment, enabling you to see past the entirety of the nerves and issues that may appear to be unconquerable. This clearness of mind will put to rest questions, and enable you to see through to the core of an issue, and to discover arrangements that you never would have seen with the chakra shut.

Sacrosanct Geometry Clothing

Advantage #6: FINDING THE BEST PATH

Attempting to make sense of where to go from where you are is one of life's endless battles. Also, in light of the fact that everybody is attempting to head off to some place unique, there is nobody answer that will work for everybody. Be that as it may, by opening your third eye, you can see inside yourself, and locate your very own way. By observing the concealed world around you, and the shrouded world withing yourself, you will get yourself, your needs, and your wants more completely than you did previously. This will enable you to settle on better choices for yourself, and to discover the open doors you have to get you from where you are, to where you need to be.

Advantage #7: LUCID DREAMING AND ASTRAL TRAVEL

Have you at any point been in a fantasy, and realized you were dreaming, however despite everything you couldn't change the course of what was going on? All things considered, there are a few people who can assume responsibility for their fantasies, and keep up their office during these nighttime experiences. This is called clear dreaming, and the individuals who are in line with their ajna chakra frequently discover they have essentially more authority over their fantasies than they did before they opened it up. There are additionally some who accept that the opening of the third eye is the way to astral travel and projection. The thought is that, by associating your psyche to the more noteworthy universe surrounding you, your awareness can leave your body to encounter different occasions and different spots.

There are a wide range of advantages to figuring out how to open your third eye chakra. It causes you become more in line with yourself, and with your general surroundings, notwithstanding enabling you to shed pressure and discover make ways to the arrangements you need in your life. While it takes a ton of work to arrive at that chakra, when you at last figure out how proportional that summit, it is all worth the exertion.

At the point when you open your third eye or enact your pineal organ, it raises the degree of understanding and instinct in you.

Your degree of cognizance increments. You can see the inconspicuous.

You more likely than not found out about "Third Eye" in Hindu folklores (otherwise called Anja, Brow or chakra). The incomparable Lord Shiva used to open his third eye when he was irate and consumed things into debris.

So don't get befuddled when gotten some information about your eyes and their tally. "Two" as an answer would not be right as in your "third eye" is the most dominant piece of your body that has genuine reality.

It is anything but a recognition yet sheer truth. In present day times, it implies edification, pre-acknowledgment, and opportunity from out-world encounters.

Chapter by chapter guide

What Is Third Eye?

How To Open Your Third Eye?

Advantages Of Awakening Third Eye

Legendary Pineal Gland

Steps To Care About The Pineal Gland

What Is Third Eye?

What Is Third Eye

What Is Third Eye

Your third eye is constantly accessible however undetectable, in contrast to our different eyes.

It gives us understanding, information, and knowledge about what occurred before, what is right now continuous in the present and what will happen later on.

It goes about as an instinct for example it sees the obscure, inconspicuous and feels unfelt. Have you at any point been abruptly halted by your mom from taking your bicycle out? This is her instinct that is only her third eye vitality. This power originates from her higher component of adoration and commitment towards you. This factor is known as the "intuition."

You may once in a while wind up viewed by somebody or may feel the nearness of somebody despite your good faith. This is only reality, which manages the nearness of spirits around you.

I won't go that far inside as certain individuals may get frightened, yet one thing without a doubt is that your "third eye" makes their quality felt.

The things you need to know are as of now dependent on you. You simply need a kick to take it out. Reflection can be that wellspring of punch, giving you a specific way to saddle that vitality. You don't need to visit your Psychic or rely upon your zodiac sign. Simply attempt to get to your instinct through profound contemplation.

The man is constantly held together by his every day ideals of feelings and stress. Attempt to control them through your cognizance that will assist you with becoming self-assured and self-controlled about your mindfulness aptitudes. This will build up your 'sense' and 'sight'. When you become mindful of your knowledge, you'll attempt to grow them.

Propelled cognizance, makes the world a little spot. Reflection encourages you in getting cognizant as well as grows new interests inside you. You can without much of a stretch arrangement with all progressing natural pressures, and your nerves will diminish bit by bit. This will make you a "man on the mission".

Another third eye magnificence is that it smothers your negative considerations and thinking. It's in human instinct to be stressed and on edge over the assignments to finish. This outcomes in negative musings. Be that as it may, when it goes, a clean cognizant vitality has its spot. This can be accomplished with standard contemplation.

The third eye encourages you to dispose of terrible minds and ambiguous dreams. Individuals constantly will in general long for things that they are directly managing; a lower vibration can make these fantasies terrible and uncertain.

Anything about your way of life, relationship, employment, and objectives can give you bad dreams whenever left unanswered. Be that as it may, they can be maintained a strategic distance from with 'third eye' for example with an unmistakable vision through reflection.

How To Open Your Third Eye?

The most effective method to OPEN YOUR THIRD EYEHOW TO OPEN YOUR THIRD EYE

The most effective method to OPEN YOUR THIRD EYE

Your third eye is symbolized by the shading 'indigo.' It is available between the foreheads and related with time and light.

Eat dull pale blue natural products, fluids, and flavors; wear purple garments to get the vibe of your third eye Start pondering and attempt to make yourself without a care in the world.

I will clarify you a basic advance to open your "third eye."

Sit in a quiet room where no clamor impact can reach.

Close your eyes and gradually attempt to feel your inward breath and exhalation to quiet your nerves.

While breathing in, carry your concentration to a specific vitality structure.

Presently center this vitality around the third eye chakra.

Start envisioning a purple chunk of vitality which becomes greater and greater with each inhales, at the area of your third eye.

Discharge all your negative considerations, nerves, dread and stress while breathing out.

Proceed till you feel yourself light and free from every single common fascination, bringing about warmth in the middle of the foreheads.

When you feel this glow, your third eye opens.

The Essence of the Sixth Chakra (Ajna): Clarity, Truth, and Unity

Regularly alluded to as the house the "third eye," the 6th chakra (otherwise called ajna chakra) is the place instinct and extraordinary awareness take need over common rationale. At the point when this 6th chakra focus is open, you can see unmistakably into another's essence—or into your own—with a knowingness that rises above the need to talk about truth or shrewdness. The third eye chakra additionally encourages you sense the vibrational flows and fundamental substratum of situational powers.

At the point when this limit is animated, you can perceive how past bearings impact present decisions and the future possibilities toward which they are pointing. Thinking, mind, suddenness, and mental adaptability all become exceptionally created at this superconscious level where you can recognize what substances appear to be and what they genuinely are. With the third eye chakra you rise above typical capacities and can see into others, life circumstances, and yourself.

Right business and truth steer the spirit's rudder of an individual living from the advanced consciousness of the 6th chakra. For the individuals who walk this way, all inclusive messages of higher realities are the focal point through which they see life and explain their discernments. Some portion of this condition of cognizant third eye chakra arousing is having the option to perceive what is valuable and accommodating to mankind and different creatures and what is hurtful—to whom for sure, when, and in what explicit ways. Utilizing this ajna chakra mindfulness valuably is the pearl of right work that is regularly seen as a significant part of an otherworldly way.

6th Chakra (Ajna) Correspondences

Key expressions: Intuition, reflective and mindfulness, mental and passionate lucidity, truth; joins knowing, acting, and feeling; balances and coordinates "manly" and "ladylike" characteristics

Physical area: The point between the eyebrows, focal point of temple

Endocrine organ: Pituitary or pineal organ (light-touchy; directs resting and waking)

Celestial connection: Saturn

Day of the week: Saturday

Component: mahat, the pith of every other component

Sense: Intuition

Sanskrit Derivation: ajna (request, order)

Back rub: Forehead, ears, sides of head among eyes and ears

Additionally, the third eye chakra is frequently called the abode of the thoughtful personnel. It epitomizes the mantra hamsa, which is Sanskrit for "swan," a worshipped fledgling that is said to have the option to recognize truth from misrepresentation as it flies to places that customary individuals can't reach. Similarly as nobody can see power or microwaves, or similarly as a canine or deer can hear numerous sounds that no human ear can hear, the unpretentious inside murmur of this mantra goes unheard by the numerous who live for the most part in their lower chakras. In any case, an ace of this ajna chakra focus who practices right job can go past the breaking points of coherent idea. By reflecting on the 6th chakra and opening the third eye and brain to the widespread characteristics of the snare of life that connections all creatures, an individual stands on the edge of the entry of celestial unity where the person in question can turn into a paramahamsa—one who abides in incomparable awareness.

Find ground-breaking bits of knowledge and systems for making brilliant wellbeing, joy, flourishing, harmony and stream in your life and connections.

For the vast majority, advancement of 6th chakra limits regularly happens along a continuum of development. Such improvement takes various structures relying upon every individual's picked way. A couple of individuals are normally arranged to the advancement of third eye chakra powers, however the majority of us need to rehearse reflective strategies to liberate the psyche from common ties and work truly to stir our lethargic ajna chakra potential to encounter the endowment of utilizing more than our five detects.

6th Chakra Abilities and Possibilities

Chances to Awaken Ajna Chakra and Positive Use of Abilities

+ Uses instinct, third eye opens

+ Feels unity with others

+ Hears others

+ Perceives totality of life

+ Sees, hears, and faculties possess internal

+ Alert and mindful

+ Hears messages from possess body

+ Taps into profound internal astuteness

+ Uses bits of knowledge about others for

+ Deep or significant correspondences

+ Detached from pride related

+ Evolving cognizance

Deterrents to Awakening Ajna Chakra and Negative Use of Abilities

+ Resists instinct, inflexibly normal

+ Views others as totally unique

+ Hears others through claim concerns

+ Distracted by subtleties

+ Has inflexible inward dividers, self-deluding certainties

+ Dreamy, not exactly here

+ Ignores messages from claim body

+ Engages in messy reasoning, stupid activity

+ Uses experiences about others for their advantage/individual increase

+ Surface or minor correspondences

+ Ego-connection to powers (siddhis) with sense of self

+ Descending cognizance, proud

Third eye contemplation benefits

Logical proof demonstrates that third eye reflection benefits are enormous and that these advantages are undeniable and can be approved. A portion of the third eye reflection advantages can be expressed as pursues:

A person's instinct (feeling of future) increments.

It makes an individual increasingly mindful and aware of his environment.

The third eye contemplation benefits in expanded Astral travel.

It accomplishes Telepathic movements.

By rehearsing third eye contemplation one can accomplish expanded fearlessness and self-trust.

The third eye contemplation improves the otherworldly characteristics of a person.

It enables a person to comprehend the idea of the universe.

It helps in discovering answers from the environment.

By rehearsing third eye contemplation, one can improve the intensity of understanding.

The third eye contemplation benefits go past investigation, thinking, and legitimization.

The reflection helps a person in settling on better life choices.

The third eye Meditation fills in as a guide in the way of the life of a person.

The third eye contemplation benefits in the correspondence with the higher and the lower measurement.

It helps in escaping from terrible minds just as obscure dreams that one gets. Individuals ordinarily will in general long for things which they are right now managing. At the point when an individual is looked with a lower vibration, it can make such dreams awful just as uncertain.

Anything parts of a person's relationship, employment, way of life, and objectives may worry him as bad dreams in the event that they are left unanswered. However, these can be illuminated with third eye' contemplation.

One all the more third eye contemplation advantage is that by rehearsing reflection, one can stifle the negative point of view of the brain and control its working.

By accomplishing propelled awareness through third eye contemplation, the world turns into a little spot. Third eye reflection helps a person to get cognizant, yet additionally helps in growing new interests.

In this manner it very well may be seen that there are an assortment of advantages that can be gotten from third eye Meditation. By utilizing third eye Meditation, one can definitely improve an incredible nature. It helps a person in carrying on with an existence of higher request with more noteworthy consciousness of himself just as the environment.

The Sanskrit word "chakra" signifies wheel, and as indicated by yoga and Ayurveda, the body contains seven primary chakras, or wheels of vitality. The seven chakras start at the base of the spine and reach out up to the crown of the head. It's at these twirling purposes of vitality and awareness where the psyche, body, and the soul meet. The 6th chakra, known as ajna, yet additionally alluded to as the third eye, is known as the base of our instinct. Be that as it may, there's quite a lot more to it.

What's the Third Eye Chakra?

The third chakra is situated at the temples, focused somewhat over the two eyes. So it bodes well that it speaks to seeing, however not simply locate. The third eye chakra speaks to clear instinct and clear musings. At the point when the third eye is opened it takes into account more clear self reflection and profound consideration. The third eye enables us to see our internal certainties and not be misled with oneself restricting stories we let ourselves know.

Genuine Benefits of Opening the Third Eye

By opening the third eye we can start to comprehend our actual selves. That "intuition" or premonition starts in the third eye, and when it's fair and open, we can see unmistakably.

Anodea Judith, Ph.D writes in her book "Wheels of Life," the third eye chakra gives us the endowment of seeing both our internal and external universes. Also, the amount we can see relies upon how open this chakra is. The advantages of opening it up include:

Diminished pressure

Honed instinct

Acknowledgment of your motivation

Capacity to move in the direction you had always wanted

Step by step instructions to Open the Third Eye

So with regards to arriving at your objectives and having your fantasies worked out as expected, opening your third eye is the best approach to complete it, no one but you can't simply open and close it like squinting your different eyes. No, it takes work. In any case, at last, it's definitely justified even despite the exertion. Get the chance to take a shot at opening your third eye.

1. Contemplation

Not certain how to begin reflecting? Steps include:

Locate a tranquil spot with negligible interruption.

Sit leg over leg on a cushion and enable the knees to fall underneath the hips.

Set the clock on your cell phone for however long you need to contemplate.

Attempt to reflect for a couple of moments consistently. Before anything else is best for a great many people on the grounds that the brain is the least blurred.

Close the eyes and pursue your breath or pick a mantra to rehash on the breathe in and breathe out. A straightforward mantra like let go or breathe in harmony and breathe out self-restricting considerations, functions admirably.

At the point when you're contemplating, concentrate and vitality on this chakra.

In the event that considerations dominate, return to the breath and pull together your consideration on the third eye chakra.

2. Reciting

Reciting invigorates the pineal organ, the glandular framework related with the 6th chakra. Reciting invigorates this hormonal focus to discharge useful hormones that manage your enthusiastic wellbeing and keep you focused for reflection.

Start by reciting OM toward the finish of your reflection.

Play Kirtan music, call and reaction Sanskrit reciting that enables you to just track.

3. Gem Healing

As per Gaia.org, certain precious stones may animate the pineal organ including amethyst, laser quartz, moonstone, pietersite, purple sapphire, purple violet tourmaline, rhodonite, rose quality, and sodalite. Consider visiting a vitality healer who works in precious stone recuperating.

Yoga to Open Up Your Third Eye

These postures work to open up the third eye for two reasons. To start with, each of the three postures advance unwinding, which considers simpler reflection. Doing these postures before you sit to ruminate, can make your training simpler. Adjusting the breath to advance folds serves to both discharge strain and quiet down your whole vessel.

Second, these yoga represents all animate the third eye chakra found marginally over the focal point of your two eyes. Before beginning your training ensure you set a goal. Remind yourself to welcome your third eye to light the path during your training and open your instinct.

1. Remaining Forward Bend

Picture of forward overlay through Shutterstock

Breathe in, arrive at the hands over head and breathe out, crease forward at the hips.

With a slight twist in the knee, bring the hands either to cloth doll, going after inverse elbows, to hinders on the floor, or to the floor itself.

Discharge strain in the neck and shoulders and let the heaviness of your head open up any tight muscles in this piece of the body.

Inhale profoundly.

With each breathe in and breathe out, discharge somewhat more profound, bringing the brow toward the shins.

You can likewise slide the hands down the calves and curve the knees as required, with the goal that your brow arrives at your shins.

This yoga present enables the progression of blood to take advantage of the third eye chakra.